POLIO VOICES

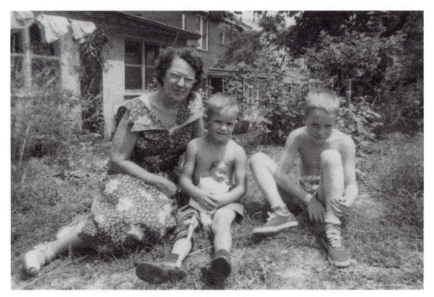

Diagnosed in 1950 with polio, Kurt Sipolski (center) is flanked by his grandmother and brother on a Virginia lawn. Photo courtesy of Kurt Sipolski.

POLIO VOICES

An Oral History from the American Polio Epidemics and Worldwide Eradication Efforts

JULIE SILVER, M.D. AND
DANIEL WILSON, PH.D.

The Praeger Series on Contemporary Health and Living

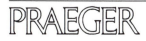

**Westport, Connecticut
London**

Library of Congress Cataloging-in-Publication Data

Silver, J. K. (Julie K.), 1965–
Polio voices : an oral history from the American polio epidemics and worldwide eradication efforts / Julie Silver and Daniel Wilson.
    p. ; cm. – (Praeger series on contemporary health and living, ISSN 1932–8079)
    Includes bibliographical references and index.
    ISBN-13: 978–0–275–99492–1 (alk. paper)
    ISBN-10: 0–275–99492–9 (alk. paper)
    1. Poliomyelitis–United States–History–20th century.   2. Poliomyelitis–Patients–United States–Interviews.
    [DNLM: 1. Poliomyelitis–history–United States.   2. Health Personnel–United States–Personal Narratives.   3. History, 20th Century–United States–Personal Narratives. 4. Poliomyelitis–United States–Personal Narratives.   5. Survivors–United States–Personal Narratives. WC 555 S587p 2007]   I. Wilson, Daniel J., 1949–   II. Title.   III. Series.
    RC181.U5S58   2007
    614.5′49–dc22   2007021464

British Library Cataloguing in Publication Data is available.

Library of Congress Catalog Card Number: 2007021464
ISBN-13: 978–0–275–99492–1
ISBN-10: 0–275–99492–9
ISSN: 1932–8079

First published in 2007

Praeger Publishers, 88 Post Road West, Westport, CT 06881
An imprint of Greenwood Publishing Group, Inc.
www.praeger.com

Printed in the United States of America

∞™

The paper used in this book complies with the Permanent Paper Standard issued by the National Information Standards Organization (Z39.48–1984).

10 9 8 7 6 5 4 3 2 1

This book is for general information only. No book can ever substitute for the judgment of a medical professional. If you have worries or concerns, contact your doctor.

Some of the names and details of individuals discussed in this book have been changed to protect the patients' identities. Some of the stories may be composites of patient interactions created for illustrative purposes.

This book is dedicated to the men and women of Rotary International who had a vision of a polio-free world and selflessly continue to work to make this dream come true.

CONTENTS

Series Foreword by Julie Silver   ix

Acknowledgments   xi

    Introduction   1

1. The Epidemic Years   15

2. Acute and Convalescent Polio   35

3. Polio's Impact on the Family   59

4. Living with Polio   75

5. The Legacy of Volunteerism   95

6. The Impact on Disability Rights in America   111

7. Post-Polio Syndrome   123

8. Polio Today and Its Effect on Advances in Medicine   139

Notes   157

Index   167

SERIES FOREWORD

Over the past hundred years, there have been incredible medical break-throughs that have prevented or cured illness in billions of people and helped many more improve their health while living with chronic conditions. A few of the most important twentieth–century discoveries include antibiotics, organ transplants, and vaccines. The twenty-first century has already heralded important new treatments including such things as a vaccine to prevent human papillomavirus from infecting and potentially leading to cervical cancer in women. Polio is on the verge of being eradicated worldwide, making it only the second infectious disease behind smallpox to ever be erased as a human health threat.

In this series, experts from many disciplines share with readers important and updated medical knowledge. All aspects of health are considered including subjects that are disease-specific and preventive medical care. Disseminating this information will help individuals to improve their health as well as researchers to determine where there are gaps in our current knowledge and policy-makers to assess the most pressing needs in health care.

Series Editor Julie Silver, M.D.
Assistant Professor
Harvard Medical School
Department of Physical Medicine and Rehabilitation

ACKNOWLEDGMENTS

With every book, there are many people who help to shepherd the project to completion. In this book, the people who should be thanked first and foremost are the ones who participated in Spaulding Rehabilitation Hospital's Polio Oral History Project. These individuals were wonderful about sharing their stories so that others would be able to understand what happened during the war on polio. Our heartfelt thanks go out to all of you who participated, whether your stories appear on these pages or not, you helped to shape this book. Thank you.

We also want to thank the people who supported the Polio Oral History Project. Diana Barrett, Walter Frontera, Steven Patrick, David Storto, Michael Sullivan and Judith Waterston, David and Dorothy Arnold, Helen Ford, Ken Handal, Bob and Ann Lonardo, David and Arlene Rubin, and many others who we do not have the space here to name, all had a part in making this project happen. Without your support, this book would not have been possible. We thank Professor Marc Shell of Harvard University and Professor Edward O'Donnell of the College of the Holy Cross. Joan Headley, director of Post-Polio Health International, was also a valuable resource. The library staff at Spaulding was terrific and special thanks go to Terry O'Brien, Alison Bozzi, and Meaghan Muir who greatly assisted in getting background material. Mary Alice Hanford was invaluable in assisting with the editing and manuscript preparation. We also want to thank Debbie Carvalko and her colleagues at Greenwood/Praeger.

There are several people who deserve special mention because they worked very hard gathering the oral histories and helping to research the information in this book. Anna Rubin did a fabulous job in gathering most of these stories. Anna is the polio education and outreach coordinator at Spaulding's International Rehabilitation Center for Polio, and she is very dedicated to helping polio survivors. Lori McCrohon and Kristen McCleary helped with the interviews.

We want to thank Muhlenberg College for a Faculty Summer Research Grant that provided support for writing and editing the volume.

Finally, we want to thank those individuals who lived what this book is about. There are literally thousands of people who helped to conquer polio. Some of them marched for the March of Dimes, others joined Rotary International and volunteered in the PolioPlus program and still others assisted the World Health Organization, United States Centers for Disease Control, UNICEF, and the Bill and Melinda Gates Foundation. Their contribution to making this world a better place is truly amazing.

INTRODUCTION

For much of the twentieth century, polio was a feared crippler of children, adolescents, and adults. Carefree summers became seasons of horror as the disease struck large numbers of people virtually every summer. It wasn't until the successful development and use of the vaccines in the 1950s and 1960s that Americans could finally look forward to summers without polio.

The hundreds of thousands of Americans who contracted paralytic polio faced a long and arduous rehabilitation in an attempt to rebuild paralyzed muscles and to resume their interrupted lives. Lengthy stays in isolation and rehabilitation hospitals, smelly hot packs of wet wool, grueling and often painful physical therapy, and repeated surgeries were the aftermath of acute poliomyelitis. Beginning in the late 1930s the National Foundation for Infantile Paralysis (NFIP) raised millions of dollars through their March of Dimes campaigns to fund research into the poliovirus, to develop a vaccine, and to pay for the care of those stricken. Those efforts culminated in the Salk and Sabin vaccines, which quickly brought an end to the polio epidemics in North America and in Europe. The polio epidemics left hundreds of thousands of men and women to live out their lives disabled by permanent paralysis. In other parts of the world, the World Health Organization (WHO) estimated that an additional 20 million would suffer as polio continued to kill and cripple into the first decade of the twenty-first century in spite of concerted efforts by WHO, Rotary International, and others to eradicate it.

Evidence for the existence of polio can be found in the ancient world. The image of a young man with a characteristic crippling of polio exists on an ancient Egyptian stele (1580–1350 BC). Descriptions of what could have been paralytic polio exist from the biblical era and from ancient Greece and Rome. Because there are many causes of lameness in children, the existence of poliomyelitis as a separate disease entity emerged only slowly. By the end of the eighteenth century, the first modern descriptions of what was almost certainly poliomyelitis appear in the literature.[1] During this long stretch of human history poliomyelitis was likely endemic with the poliovirus in constant circulation.

Since the poliovirus is primarily an intestinal virus and is shed in fecal material, infection occurs most frequently through contaminated food or water or from unclean hands and utensils. In the era before modern sanitation, and in parts of the developing world today, most infants are exposed to the poliovirus while maternal antibodies in breast milk protect them. Occasionally, a child who had developed no antibodies would succumb to the disease and would be left with permanent paralysis. Even in unprotected populations the poliovirus only rarely causes permanent paralysis. Indeed, during an epidemic approximately 90 percent of the cases are unapparent but capable of spreading the disease and 4 to 8 percent are abortive in which the patient has only a mild illness. Only 1 to 2 percent of cases go on to infect the central nervous system, including the spinal cord, which causes temporary or permanent paralysis and in severe cases, death.[2]

As sanitation improved in the nineteenth century and interrupted the constant circulation of the poliovirus, polio became epidemic. The first sizeable and well-documented epidemic in the United States involving 132 cases occurred around Rutland, Vermont, in 1894. Polio epidemics were also beginning to occur in northern Europe and doctors began to study this newly emergent epidemic disease. In 1908, the Vienna immunologist Karl Landsteiner and his assistant Erwin Popper discovered the poliovirus. Dr. Simon Flexner at the Rockefeller Institute in New York City soon became the leading American polio researcher.[3]

Epidemics of the disease became both more common and more serious in the early twentieth century. New York experienced epidemics in 1907 and 1911.[4] The largest epidemic in the early twentieth century occurred in New York and the northeastern United States in 1916. The epidemic recorded 27,000 cases and 6,000 deaths in twenty-six states. New York City saw 8,900 cases with 2,400 fatalities. The large number of children and adolescents permanently paralyzed and the high mortality rate created fear and panic. Doctors and public health officials tried to stop the disease by quarantining infected families, isolating victims in contagious disease hospitals, and conducting sanitation campaigns to kill flies and clean up garbage. Communities outside affected areas banned travelers fleeing the epidemic.[5] The 1916 epidemic enabled researchers to come to four conclusions about the disease: (1) polio was transmitted from person to person without an intermediate host, although the precise mechanism was not yet identified; (2) the number of individuals infected with the poliovirus who show symptoms of the disease far outnumber those who became paralyzed; (3) these unrecognized carriers and mild cases helped spread polio; and (4) that an epidemic immunizes a substantial portion of the population against future attacks.[6] Researchers, however, were no closer to finding a preventive or a cure. Over the next several decades, research revised the medical image of the disease. Doctors understood polio as "a disease of cleanliness, occurring only among children who had been protected in early infancy from polio infection." They recognized that polio was not "primarily a disease of the central nervous system but a systemic infection centered in the intestines." After poliovirus was discovered in sewage, researchers acknowledged the presence of "widespread hidden infection."[7] Because medicine had no means to prevent the disease or paralysis, polio remained a feared crippler.

The public image of polio changed after 1921 when a rising young politician from New York, Franklin D. Roosevelt, contracted polio at the age of thirty-nine.[8] Although well beyond the usual age of polio victims, Roosevelt's social and economic status had left him unprotected against what was commonly called infantile paralysis. Polio left Roosevelt with permanently paralyzed legs. Because Roosevelt still harbored political ambitions, the full extent of his disability was concealed.[9] Roosevelt worked hard to rehabilitate his weakened and paralyzed muscles and to learn to walk once again. In 1924 at the urging of a friend Roosevelt visited the naturally heated pools at a run-down resort in Warm Springs, Georgia. The warm water facilitated his exercises and helped him move his paralyzed limbs. After a reporter publicized Roosevelt's successful visit, other polio survivors traveled to Warm Springs in hopes of recovery. In 1926 Roosevelt purchased the resort and turned it into a center for polio rehabilitation. He established the Georgia Warm Springs Foundation in 1927 to raise funds to improve the facilities and to provide care for polio patients. Warm Springs soon became a Mecca for polio survivors.[10]

After Roosevelt became president of the United States in 1933, he became a model for many polio survivors.[11] In addition, Roosevelt lent his support to efforts to raise funds for polio research and the rehabilitation of polio survivors. From 1934 to 1938 a series of Birthday Balls were organized on Roosevelt's birthday to raise money for Warm Springs. Roosevelt supported the establishment of the National Foundation for Infantile Paralysis (NFIP) in 1938 under the leadership of Basil O'Connor. The National Foundation with its March of Dimes fund-raising campaigns quickly became the major supporter of medical research into the disease and of funding to care for polio patients.[12] Between 1938 and 1959 the National Foundation raised over $622 million and spent $315 million on polio care, $55 million on research, and $33 million on educating health professionals.[13] This fund-raising set new standards and its methods were soon emulated by other organizations. During these years the government provided almost no money for medical research, most Americans lacked health and hospital insurance, and governments provided medical care only for the truly indigent. The National Foundation clearly hastened the end of the polio epidemics and softened the blow on those who had polio. Although the search for a vaccine was agonizingly slow, several medical developments improved the lives of polio patients and reduced their mortality. In 1928, Philip Drinker, an engineer at Harvard Medical School, developed the first successful tank respirator, or iron lung. The value of iron lungs in cases of respiratory paralysis soon became evident. Shortly after the NFIP was established it began to purchase iron lungs and distribute them around the country. In the early 1950s the NFIP established regional respirator centers to conduct research on respirator therapy, to train therapists in using respirators, and to treat complicated cases. These centers made it possible for many respirator-dependent patients to go home.[14]

Although the development of iron lungs was dramatic, the methods of treating polio developed by an Australian bush nurse were probably more significant for most polio survivors. Sister Elizabeth Kenny had developed a treatment for paralysis by applying hot packs of wet wool to loosen contracted muscles followed by passive stretching and movement of paralyzed limbs. Previously, the deformities of polio had generally been treated by splinting and casting to immobilize limbs in their proper alignment. Although a reaction against immobilization had already begun before Kenny arrived in the United States in 1940, her demonstration of the success of her methods spelled the end of most casting and splinting. Sister Kenny was a controversial figure in part due to her forceful personality, in part due to her theory that paralytic polio was a muscle disease rather than a disease of the central nervous system, and in part because she rejected prevailing orthodox treatment. As a female nurse and a foreigner, Sister Kenny encountered great resistance from many American physicians. However, her methods marked a significant improvement in the treatment of polio patients. They helped restore muscle strength and her involvement of the patient in the recovery of muscle function encouraged the patient's participation in rehabilitation.[15] For polio survivors in the 1940s and 1950s, the memory of malodorous, wool hot packs, and painfully stretched muscles is almost universal.

During the late 1940s scientists made considerable progress toward developing a vaccine to prevent polio. For example, John Enders, Thomas Weller, and Frederick Robbins at Harvard succeeded in growing poliovirus in tissue cultures in the laboratory. This meant laboratories could produce enough virus to make a vaccine.[16] In the late 1940s Dr. Jonas Salk began to develop a killed-virus vaccine. Salk was not the first to develop a killed-virus vaccine but in the early 1950s he demonstrated that a killed-virus vaccine would work and he perfected the methods to produce a safe vaccine in large quantities.[17] Salk's work was supported by the NFIP and when his early trials with small populations proved safe and effective, the organization decided to conduct a mass field trial. Dr. Thomas Francis, Jr., of the University of Michigan agreed to direct a field trial in 1954 that enrolled large numbers of children to be vaccinated and a large number of controls who would not be. Over 1.8 million children in forty-four states participated in the trial either receiving the Salk vaccine or serving as controls.[18] After nearly a year of suspense, Dr. Francis announced on April 12, 1955, that the Salk vaccine was safe and effective. Francis reported it was 60 to 70 percent effective against Type I polio and over 90 percent effective against Type II and Type III.[19] The United States government licensed the Salk vaccine that afternoon. Although parents throughout the United States breathed a sigh of relief, a note of uncertainty appeared two weeks later when a number of children who had been vaccinated developed polio. Mass vaccinations were immediately suspended until it was determined that some vaccine produced by Cutter Laboratories contained live poliovirus. Ultimately 204 cases of polio and eleven deaths were associated with the bad vaccine. Once it was clear that this was an isolated incident, the mass vaccinations continued and the Salk vaccine began to reduce significantly the number of new cases of polio.[20]

While supporting the development of the Salk vaccine, the National Foundation had continued to support scientists working on an attenuated live polio vaccine. Many scientists and doctors preferred the advantages promised by a safe attenuated live vaccine. An attenuated live vaccine, such as that developed by Dr. Albert Sabin, had several advantages over a killed vaccine. The live vaccine mimicked an infection with a "wild" virus but with a virus weakened and incapable of causing polio. The immune response was also stronger. This meant that no subsequent booster doses were required. In addition, immunity developed within days rather than months, which meant that such a vaccine could be used to stop an epidemic already in progress. And finally, giving the vaccine orally on a sugar cube was easier than injecting it.[21] In spite of these advantages, there is a higher risk of vaccine-associated polio with the attenuated live polio vaccine. Sabin vaccines were tested in a number of countries in the late 1950s, but especially in the Soviet Union where a massive field trial was conducted. When these field trials proved that the Sabin vaccine was generally safe and effective, it was licensed for use in the United States in 1962 and ultimately approved for use worldwide.[22] Because of its advantages, WHO has used a Sabin-type attenuated live polio vaccine in their effort to eradicate polio worldwide.

The Salk and Sabin vaccines quickly eliminated polio as a public health threat in the United States. One of the worst polio epidemics had occurred in 1952 when 57,879 cases were reported. That is far more than the 27,000 cases in 1916, although the case rate of 37.2 per 100,000 population is below the 41.1 per 100,000 in the 1916 epidemic. In 1955, the first year the Salk vaccine was available, there were 28,985 cases. However, by 1957 there were only 5,485 cases and by 1960 only 3,190. Following the introduction of the Sabin vaccine in 1962, polio rates continued to drop. In 1962 there were 940 cases, in 1965 only 73 and by 1970 only 33. The last wild virus case occurred in 1979, and this held until 2005 when four Amish children, presumably unvaccinated, were diagnosed with polio in Minnesota. During the final decades of the twentieth century, there continued to be a few cases every year, most of which were thought to be attributed to the vaccine.[23]

The development of the polio vaccines and the near eradication of polio represent one of the triumphs of twentieth-century medicine. However, the vaccine came too late for the many thousands who had already contracted the disease. The voices of polio survivors, family members, physicians, and therapists, as well as those of people who have worked on the eradication efforts testify vividly to the widespread fear of the disease, to the distressing separation from family during long hospitalizations, to the pain of acute poliomyelitis and the often painful therapies, to the difficulties and challenges of resuming an interrupted life, and most recently to the unexpected and disturbing development of the symptoms of post-polio syndrome. These stories, which are part of a collection from the Polio Oral History Project at Spaulding Rehabilitation Hospital's International Rehabilitation Center for Polio, are sometimes overshadowed by the dramatic story of conquering polio. Yet the voices of these men and women are no less important to the story of polio than those of the doctors who found ways to prevent and eradicate the disease.

Polio often began with a fever and nausea that imitated any number of minor childhood illnesses. In most cases, the child or young adult experienced an uncomfortable summer flu for several days and then recovered. Well over 90 percent of infections were unapparent or abortive. However, in individuals where the virus left the intestinal tract and invaded the central nervous system, paralysis began to appear eight to ten days after infection and several days after the onset of illness.[24] During the years when polio was at its height (1930–1956) parents and children alike viewed the onset of illness in the summer with dread. In the absence of paralysis, polio was difficult to diagnose since its early symptoms were like many other minor illnesses. Once paralysis appeared, usually in legs or arms, doctors diagnosed polio and the patient was usually quickly sent to an isolation hospital to prevent the spread of the disease. Many polio patients were given a painful spinal tap to confirm the clinical diagnoses of polio. As paralysis spread, polio patients found themselves in the fearfully alienating setting of an isolation ward, denied the comforting presence of parents and family, and surrounded by nurses and doctors in masks and gowns to reduce their own exposure to the disease. The spread of paralysis was terrifying, and no more so than when the muscles of breathing were affected. Many polio survivors recall the whoosh-whoosh of the iron lungs on the wards, the dread with which they were viewed, and the welcome relief they provided when one's breathing failed. Acute paralytic poliomyelitis was both physically and emotionally painful as individuals were rapidly transformed into partially or wholly paralyzed polio patients.

Once the crisis of acute poliomyelitis passed and they were no longer infectious, patients were moved to rehabilitation facilities. Here began the painful and all too slow rehabilitation of weakened muscles. Most polio patients endured Kenny hot packs in rehabilitation until physicians determined that maximum extension of contracted muscles had been achieved. Long stays in the rehabilitation facilities were common. While some may have gone home after only a few weeks, others remained for months, sometimes years. The rehabilitation wards were typically age and sex segregated. Some hospitals were also racially segregated, especially in the South. Polio patients often formed communities on the wards. Ward mates supported one another emotionally, encouraged friends to continue painful exercises, found ways to entertain themselves, complained about hospital regulations and food, pulled pranks on one another and the nurses, and planned for their release. No polio rehabilitation was easy, but those dependent on iron lungs faced particular challenges in being weaned from their dependence on the respirator. These long hospitalizations marked only the beginning of recovery from polio, which usually continued upon returning home.

A case of paralytic polio affected the entire family. Parents whose children contracted polio often felt guilty that they had not protected them. Perhaps they had let their son go swimming, or allowed their daughter to go on a sleepover with friends a few days before the illness began. Children and adolescents sometimes felt they had brought the disease on themselves when they had disobeyed their parents' warnings and admonitions. Families feared the stigma of having a polio patient in their midst and some families were ostracized by neighbors when polio was diagnosed. Parents often spent long hours and days at the hospital, even if they could view their child only through a window. Other children in the family sometimes felt abandoned because their parents' attention was directed toward the sick child. The families of adult polio patients faced other problems. When the husband was stricken, the family's income often ended. Worries about hospital and doctor bills only added to the concern about the loss of income. When the wife contracted polio, families worried about managing the household and caring for the children. Few families had hospital or medical insurance, so the substantial cost of polio care worried all but the wealthiest families.[25] While the National Foundation paid for the care of many polio patients, and other assistance was sometimes available, polio, nonetheless, placed a substantial financial burden on families.[26]

While going home was eagerly anticipated, the transition to home, family, school, and work was not always smooth. Houses and apartments were not usually accessible, and adjustments had to be made to accommodate the mobility limitations of the returning family member. After a lengthy hospitalization, the polio survivor had to relearn the give and take of family life from an altered perspective. Other family members had to adjust as well. There were many things polio survivors could not do, depending on the extent of their paralysis. Survivors who returned home still dependent on respirator assistance required substantial care from family members. Most families, however, eventually found ways to reintegrate the polio survivor into the ongoing life of the family, but not without some difficulty.

Even after they returned home, many polio survivors faced continuing physical therapy or surgery to correct deformities. Family members often took on the daily task of providing hot packs to reduce pain and enhance flexibility. Fathers sometimes constructed exercise equipment to strengthen muscles. Other polio survivors had daily outpatient therapy at Easter Seals or similar facilities. Many had returned home using braces, which required alteration and adjustment. Polio survivors often faced additional hospitalizations after their initial homecoming. Doctors generally waited at least two years after polio to ascertain how much function could be regained through therapy. However, if deformities remained, many physicians recommended corrective surgery. These occurred anywhere from three to ten years after polio and required additional, sometimes lengthy, hospitalizations. For adolescent survivors summers often meant not carefree vacations but another return to the operating room, more pain, and additional therapy. Spinal fusions to correct scoliosis were the most dramatic and involved long confinements in body casts to straighten the spine and to protect the fused vertebrae. Full recovery from polio thus sometimes stretched for years before doctors decided that no more medical interventions were necessary.

Resuming one's life after polio was challenging. Children and adolescents had to become part of the family, classroom, and neighborhood once again. Husbands and wives, mothers and fathers, had to learn how to be a spouse and parent on crutches or from a wheelchair or iron lung. Children and adolescents worried about keeping up with their class and returning to school. Most survivors did return successfully, although they often had to negotiate inaccessible buildings, deal with unsupportive teachers and schoolyard taunts, struggle through physical education, and sit on the sidelines of sporting events. Others, because the schools were inaccessible or their impairments were too severe, were taught at home. Adult survivors were anxious to return to work both as a validation of their self-worth and for the income. Fortunately, some employers had kept their jobs open until they could return. That return, of course, was predicated on their ability to continue to do the work. Others faced the challenge of finding new jobs, either because their former employer had replaced them or because their impairments precluded returning to their former employment. Many polio survivors found it difficult to convince employers that in fact they were good workers even though they used braces or a wheelchair. Although they faced numerous challenges, polio survivors are notable for their high levels of education and employment.[27]

Polio survivors as a group have lived remarkably successful lives. Significant numbers of them finished their schooling, married, had children, and enjoyed successful careers. Many had taken to heart the Protestant work ethic reinforced during their polio rehabilitation: hard persistent effort pursued over a long time brought significant rewards. That ethic had carried polio survivors through painful therapies. Many polio survivors applied then that same principle to the challenges they faced in gaining an education, raising a family, and succeeding at work. Polio survivors pushed their bodies to enable them to succeed in spite of the obstacles. That was how they had beaten polio initially, and it was a lesson that stayed with them for a lifetime.

Many survivors were told that once they achieved maximum physical recovery they could expect a long period of stability. No one warned them about the late effects of polio: muscle pain, weakness, and fatigue. No one prepared them for post-polio syndrome. Although scattered medical articles from the early twentieth century noted the late effects of polio, they were overlooked when polio was at its peak.[28] However, by the late 1970s when the large mid-century cohort of polio survivors entered their third decade of living with their impairments, many, to their dismay and distress, began to experience the now familiar symptoms. They could no longer walk as far. Muscles tired more easily and the pain of overexertion increased. When they consulted their current physicians, many of whom were unfamiliar with polio, they often found no answers. Indeed, doctors attributed the problems to growing older, stress, or an overactive imagination. Polio survivors, many of them working through the network established by Gini Laurie, the Gazette International Networking Institute, pushed for medical recognition of the perplexing symptoms. GINI first sponsored a conference on the late effects of polio in 1981. Since then they have sponsored eight more conferences, the last in 2005, bringing together polio survivors, physicians, scientists, and therapists in an effort to understand the causes of the symptoms and to explore ways of alleviating them.[29] The publication of good advice manuals has helped polio survivors understand and cope with post-polio syndrome.[30]

Post-polio syndrome has had a significant impact on the lives of many polio survivors. Men and women suddenly found themselves unable to function in their day-to-day lives. Some had to seek flexible work schedules or a less strenuous position. Others had to apply for disability benefits or retire early. Women who had run the household found that they now needed assistance with their daily chores. Steps now became obstacles. Breathing became more difficult. Individuals who had risen out of their wheelchairs to walk with braces and crutches found themselves reliant once again on a wheelchair for mobility. Others had to move to a powered chair. Many polio survivors have experienced the symptoms of post-polio as a second disability, often with significant psychological and emotional consequences.[31] If the advice of therapists in the forties and fifties was "use it or lose it," the advice to polio survivors today is "use it and lose it." But it has been difficult to turn away from the beliefs and habits that helped polio survivors succeed at so much and to reconfigure their beliefs and practices so that doing more with less becomes the new measure of success.

The legacy of the polio epidemics extends well beyond its impact on the individuals who contracted the disease. The polio epidemics and the ways in which Americans responded to them created a legacy that eventually affected attitudes toward and treatment of individuals with disabilities. These responses also changed volunteerism, fund-raising, and patient advocacy, and brought new advances in medicine. Inspired by the model of Franklin D. Roosevelt, polio survivors since the 1930s have expected to fulfill their dreams of an education, a family, and a career. When physical and attitudinal barriers have blocked them, polio survivors fought individually and collectively to eliminate them. Many of the individuals who created and who have led the disability rights movement in this country have been polio survivors. The NFIP set new standards and practices for fund-raising, for funding basic research into the disease and into developing a successful vaccine, and for providing patient care. Volunteerism and the efforts of private foundations, especially Rotary International, have been crucial to the effort to eliminate polio throughout the world. Polio survivors, along with disabled veterans, pushed for improved methods of rehabilitation, better assistive devices including braces, wheelchairs, respirators, and ventilators, and for returning the disabled to active lives in the community. Polio survivors had many allies as they shaped their legacy, including their families, many physicians and therapists, and other disabled men and women, but there is no doubt that they played an important role in reshaping treatment of the disabled in the last half of the twentieth century.

Polio survivors often believed that they could accomplish anything they wanted in spite of the limitations imposed by the disease. Polio rehabilitation influenced by the example of Warm Springs and Sister Kenny emphasized rebuilding strength and function so survivors could return to home, school, and work. Many homes were modified to accommodate polio survivors' needs, but where they were not survivors typically made do. When schools were inaccessible, survivors and their parents pressed school boards and principals to make accommodations. With their education in hand, polio survivors struggled to enter the workforce, and most eventually did in spite of inaccessible workplaces and skeptical employers. In the 1960s and 1970s polio survivors began to articulate the idea of disability rights and to demand full access. Ed Roberts and others at the University of California Berkeley in the 1960s forced the university to admit them, to provide access to classes and other activities, and to provide the support they needed to be independent. They also pressured state departments of vocational rehabilitation to fund independent living. The efforts of Roberts and others eventually gave rise to the independent living movement to enable all individuals with disabilities to live as independently as possible.[32] The architect Ron Mace became a leading figure in the universal design movement that emphasizes designing for accessibility for all types of disabilities.[33] And polio survivors like Justin Dart, Jr., lobbied extensively to build support for the Americans with Disabilities Act.[34] Polio survivors have played a key role in pushing to make the United States accessible for all.

From the late 1920s on volunteer organizations have been in the forefront of the efforts to find a cure for polio, to care for those stricken by the disease and, ultimately, to eradicate it completely. The first of these was the Georgia Warm Springs Foundation established by Franklin D. Roosevelt in 1927 to support the polio rehabilitation facility he had created. In 1933 the President's Birthday Ball Commission was established to raise additional funds for the fight against polio.[35]

In 1938, Basil O'Connor and Roosevelt announced the formation of the NFIP with three goals: raising funds to provide medical care to all polio patients, educating the public about polio, and raising funds to support research into the disease and to find a cure.[36] The entertainer Eddie Cantor coined the phrase March of Dimes and Americans were asked to send their dimes to the White House. The total receipts were over $1.8 million. Fifty percent of the funds were returned to local NFIP chapters to be used for polio care in their communities. The other half went toward research and administrative expenses. The foundation established a Committee on Scientific Research to evaluate research proposals and to make grants in support of the research.[37] The NFIP came on the scene at a time when the polio researchers were poised to make significant advances against the disease, but the ultimate successes against polio would not have come as quickly without the help of the National Foundation.[38] Between 1938 and 1955, the National Foundation devoted $203.6 million to patient care and $22.6 million to research[39] In the widespread use of volunteers, in the innovative fund-raising techniques developed, in the combination of funding patient care and scientific research, in the total dollars raised, and in the ultimate success of the Salk and Sabin vaccines, the NFIP set new standards for health-related volunteer organizations.

The dramatic success of the Salk vaccine prompted the National Foundation in the late 1950s to reassess its purpose. The National Foundation turned away from polio and focused on reducing birth defects and infant mortality.[40] Volunteerism, however, still had a role to play in worldwide polio eradication efforts. Beginning in 1985 Rotary International, a voluntary organization with chapters in 160 countries, initiated its PolioPlus program to raise funds in support of WHO's campaign to eliminate polio.[41] Rotary International has raised over 600 million dollars for the campaign, and inspired other groups to help fund the effort.[42] By 2005 polio had been eliminated in all but a few countries in Africa and Asia. Worldwide the number of cases of polio had dropped to 1,266 in 2004.[43]

Another legacy of the polio epidemics was improvements in rehabilitative practices and in assistive devices. The large number of polio patients requiring rehabilitation at mid-century encouraged the development of new techniques to strengthen muscles, restore function, and develop modes of compensation. The iron lung was one of the first successful respirators and quickly became an iconic image of the epidemics. The proven success of the iron lungs also encouraged the development of smaller and less cumbersome methods of ventilation.[44] The sheer numbers of polio patients requiring bracing and dependent on wheelchairs also encouraged the development of lighter and more effective devices. The physical needs of this large cohort of patients and their determination to return to their homes and communities fostered innovations in rehabilitative techniques and assistive devices.

Polio Voices presents the stories of men and women who had polio decades ago. Participants in the Polio Oral History Project volunteered to be interviewed about their experience with polio from the time of diagnosis to the development of post-polio syndrome. We have also included interviews from healthcare providers and people who have participated in the polio eradication effort. Although interviewers had a carefully developed set of questions, they were also flexible in letting the participants tell their own stories. The polio accounts set down in this volume are lightly edited transcripts of the taped interviews.

Although a few of the polio survivors had journals, letters, or scrapbooks to jog their memories, many of the interviewees relied solely on their vivid memories. How truthful are these memories recorded several decades after the events they described occurred? Recent scholarship in psychology and on illness narratives supports the fundamental veracity of these stories, even if individuals may have forgotten some of the details. Acute polio and the long rehabilitation that typically followed were traumatic for many patients regard-less of their age when they contracted the disease. *Remembering Trauma*, a recent work by Richard J. McNally, professor of psychology at Harvard, re-views a considerable body of experimental and clinical research on memory and on the memory of trauma. McNally argues that all the evidence suggests that "autobiographical recollection is a reconstructive, not reproductive, pro-cess." Not all the details of the original experience were encoded in the brain, nor does the individual always recall all the details that were encoded. How-ever, McNally argues that "memory for the gist of many experiences is retained with essential fidelity, and this is especially true for events having personal, emotional significance," which the experience of acute polio, paralysis, and subsequent rehabilitation certainly was.[45] These recent studies thus support the likelihood that polio survivors of all ages retain vivid memories of their polio experience even if some of the details have become blurred or forgotten.

Scholars who have studied the flourishing genre of illness and disability narratives in recent decades have come to similar conclusions concerning the essential truthfulness of these accounts. Anne Hunsaker Hawkins, for example, argues that what she calls "pathographies" may indeed be read as "true stories," but the emphasis must be as much on the word "stories" as the word "true." She writes that "to emphasize the 'story' element in these narratives is in no way to denigrate their truth-value." Hawkins concludes that "the process of autobiographical recollection is part self-discovery and part self-creation."[46]

Arthur Frank has also explored the truthfulness of what he calls illness stories. He acknowledges that "the stories we tell about our lives are not necessarily those lives as they were lived, but these stories become our expe-rience of those lives." He notes that stories about illness can change over a lifetime: "Life moves on, stories change with that movement, and experience changes." Frank argues that "the truth of stories is not only what *was* experi-enced, but equally what *becomes* experience in the telling and its reception." The stories told in this volume don't always conform to the popular image of dedicated physicians, hardworking compassionate nurses, and polio survivors who through hard work and determination triumphed over their impairments. But, as Frank observes, "what makes an illness story good is the act of witness that says, implicitly or explicitly, 'I will tell you not what you want to hear but what I know to be true because I have lived it.'"[47] In telling of lives shaped by polio and its aftermath, these survivors often acknowledge that one doesn't so much triumph over polio as learn to live with it and to adjust to the disease's long-term impact on their bodies and their lives.

Polio Voices, then, allows us to hear what it was like to contract a greatly feared childhood disease, to experience spreading paralysis, to undergo an arduous recovery and rehabilitation, and to encounter obstacles and discrim-ination on attempting to resume one's interrupted life. But the volume also gives voice to those who cared for polio patients in isolation hospitals and on rehabilitation wards, to those who developed the equipment that allowed polio survivors to return to home, school, and work, to those who conducted the research that eventually brought an end to polio in the United States and, potentially, the world, and to those who raised the funds to support the medical and scientific research and the polio care that made all this possible. The polio epidemics are a rapidly fading memory in the United States, and, with hard work and a little luck, will soon be eradicated worldwide. But the threat of epidemic disease remains real. One only has to think of the infectious diseases that have emerged since polio's decline including HIV/AIDS, West Nile Virus, and avian flu. And of course, the more recent threat of bioterrorism only heightens the concern. Thus, it is important to remember what it was like to live with summers of fear when children and young adults were permanently paralyzed by an unseen virus and medicine was for a long time helpless to stop the epidemic from spreading. But if the polio epidemics remind us of a fearful time, they should also remind us of what the human spirit is capable. Hundreds of thousands of men, women, and children raised funds that provided medical care for the stricken and for research that eventually led to a cure. Thousands of doctors and nurses risked their own health and that of their families to care for acutely ill polio patients. And hundreds of thousands of individuals who contracted polio demonstrated real courage and determination in working hard to rehabilitate their paralyzed bodies and to resume lives so abruptly altered by the disease. Polio would prove to have a lifelong impact on those who had the disease, but polio survivors have been resilient and the strong voices in this volume are testimony to that resilience and determination.

1

THE EPIDEMIC YEARS

Beginning in the late nineteenth century, Americans had a new reason to fear summers: polio. In the summer of 1894 in the vicinity of Rutland, Vermont, the largest polio epidemic yet seen in America occurred. Dr. Charles S. Caverly described an epidemic that involved 132 cases. This epidemic had several noteworthy features: Caverly observed that increasingly older children were becoming ill with polio and that six of the patients had all the nervous system signs of polio but no paralysis. Both features became prominent during the twentieth-century epidemics. The next substantial epidemic in the United States occurred in New York City in 1907 when over 750 cases were reported.[1] Polio was also in the news in 1908 when the Viennese scientist Karl Landsteiner and his assistant Erwin Popper discovered the virus that caused polio.[2] Thus, within fifteen years of the first notable epidemic in the United States polio had begun to garner significant medical attention. However, it took the 1916 epidemic in New York and the northeast to impress the fear of polio on the American public.

Twenty-six states in the northeastern United States reported over 27,000 cases with 6,000 deaths. New York City saw 8,900 cases and nearly one child in four (2,400) who became ill died. Although polio cases were reported as far west as Kansas and Wisconsin, the Mid-Atlantic States were hit the hardest. Public health authorities tried to stem the epidemic through quarantines and the isolation of children with the disease, banning public gatherings and closing schools, and campaigns advocating cleanliness and elimination of the flies.[3]

As Naomi Rogers argues in her fine study of the 1916 polio epidemic, "polio appeared particularly strange and frightening because of physicians' and the public's high expectations of science and scientists." Polio's epidemic appearance "struck a jarring note in this time of scientific optimism" because so little was known about the disease and because medicine could neither prevent it nor stop the spread of paralysis once begun. Polio called into question strategies that had begun to decrease the awful toll of infectious diseases. In addition, "polio epidemics also contradicted traditional models of disease transmission: polio cases appeared in both overcrowded slums and sparsely populated suburbs.... Its victims were often children who were previously healthy, well nourished, and protected."[4]

Even during the devastating epidemic of 1916, when the rate was 41.1 per 100,000 population, polio occurred far less often than other serious infectious diseases that sickened and killed thousands every year. As late as 1930, tuberculosis infected 101.5 of every 100,000 Americans and killed 70 of every 100,000.[5] In 1916, other childhood diseases and killers all had much higher incidence rates than polio.[6] And two years after the polio epidemic had shocked New York and the nation, the great influenza epidemic of 1918–1919 killed about 550,000 in the United States, almost 25,000 in New York City, and an estimated twenty million worldwide.[7] Why then did polio have such a dramatic effect in 1916 and subsequently? In part it was because epidemic polio appeared to be a new disease that modern medicine did not understand and could not prevent or cure. The other major diseases of childhood were equally devastating, but their very familiarity reduced their social and cultural impact. Parents, in particular, feared polio's ability to cripple not only their child's body, but also his or her chances to find a job, to marry, and to succeed in life.

Following the great 1916 epidemic, polio returned to relatively low levels of incidence. However, a single case of polio in 1921, that of Franklin D. Roosevelt, helped keep the disease in the public mind. Roosevelt's recovery and his efforts on behalf of polio rehabilitation became frequent subjects in the national media.[8] As Rogers observed, "the experience of one of America's most famous polio sufferers . . . did much to transform the public perception of the disease. No longer solely associated with poor immigrants, polio had struck a wealthy young man and created a cripple" who, nonetheless, went on to win two prominent political offices.[9]

During the 1930s polio generally remained at relatively low levels of incidence nationally, although several serious local epidemics, such as the 1934 Los Angeles epidemic received considerable attention.[10] Roosevelt's election helped shape the cultural impact of polio in several ways. Thousands of polio patients and their families wrote President Roosevelt seeking encouragement and reassurance as they struggled with the disease.[11] Roosevelt also became associated with a national effort to raise funds to support polio rehabilitation and research leading to effective means to prevent or cure polio.[12]

Polio also came to public attention in a less positive fashion in the 1930s when two physicians who had been working separately on developing a vaccine, Drs. Maurice Brodie and John A. Kolmer, conducted unsuccessful human trials that resulted in several cases of vaccine-induced polio. Both vaccine trials were quickly stopped and "the disastrous results of these early efforts were sufficient to dampen any further attempts to immunize man for a dozen or more years."[13] In spite of this spectacular failure, physicians were finally beginning to make real progress in understanding the poliovirus and the recurrent epidemics.

In 1937, Roosevelt and his advisors decided to create a national organization to conduct fund-raising on behalf of polio patients and polio research. Basil O'Connor became the president of the National Foundation for Infantile Paralysis (NFIP) when it was established early in 1938. The singer Eddie Cantor coined the phrase "March of Dimes" while suggesting that citizens send their dimes to the White House in support of this new effort to fight polio. The White House mailroom received 2,680,000 dimes as well other coins, bills, and checks.[14] Although physicians were uncomfortable with the advertising and public relations approach to raising funds, they were grateful for the research monies the NFIP provided.[15] The NFIP, aided by its association with President Roosevelt, soon made polio and the conquest of the disease a national issue. As John Paul noted, "the effective use of propaganda techniques" created "public interest in poliomyelitis research as a holy quest. The image of the disease as an evil thing that must be conquered and banished forevermore took hold."[16]

The very success of the NFIP significantly changed the experience of polio. Most importantly, care and treatment improved when the National Foundation began paying for many, although not all, polio patients. In addition, some of the NFIP monies went to train nurses and doctors in new, more effective procedures. Polio survivors, especially local and national poster children, were held up as heroes who triumphed over their disease and disabilities with the help of the freely given dimes. But there was another side to all the publicity efforts of the NFIP to educate Americans about polio and to encourage donations. The posters of cute kids in braces and wheelchairs, the displays of iron lungs in department stores, the dramatic news accounts of the summer epidemics all fanned fear of the disease.

Polio care was also changing in the thirties and forties. Two developments, in particular, deserve mention—the iron lung and the therapeutic methods of Sister Elizabeth Kenny. Although there were some dramatic early cases in which the lives of polio patients were saved because of an available iron lung, doctors were generally cautious in their enthusiasm for the device. In spite of fairly high early mortality rates, the iron lungs gradually became a common tool to fight polio, especially once the NFIP began to pay for treatment. By 1940 between four and five hundred children were treated in iron lungs every year. Iron lungs were expensive, costing between $2,000 and $3,000 in the forties.[17] New patients in polio hospitals viewed with dread the large yellow tanks sitting silently in the hall or a corner of the ward. But if their breathing muscles were paralyzed, and they struggled for every breath, the yellow monsters suddenly became their angels, allowing them to breathe easily once again. Only a small percentage of polio patients ever needed an iron lung, and most who were dependent on them would recover enough to eventually breathe on their own or with the aid of other devices, such as a rocking bed, but throughout the polio epidemics the prospect of being entombed in an iron lung was among the greatest fears.

Beginning in the mid-1940s, the vast majority of patients afflicted with the paralytic polio experienced the Sister Kenny method of treatment, or some version of her procedures. Polio was capricious in the nerves it weakened or destroyed, often leaving one of a pair of muscles atrophied or significantly weaker. The result was the characteristic contractures of polio, which could twist arms, legs, and torsos into grotesque and painful shapes. Before the 1940s the typical treatment was to encase the affected body parts in plaster casts to prevent the contractures. It was not unusual for patients to spend months in such casts.

With Kenny's methods the disfiguring and disabling contractures would be eliminated or at least lessened and the polio patient would gradually move from assisted movement of the muscles to moving them on her/his own. Her methods of treating acute and convalescent polio patients soon became commonplace. John Paul believed that "Sister Kenny's ideas and techniques marked a turning point, even an about-face, in the aftercare of paralytic poliomyelitis. By determination and sheer willpower she helped to raise the treatment of paralyzed patients out of the slough into which it had sunk in the 1930s."[18]

The characteristics of the polio epidemics in the forties and fifties were also changing. For reasons that are not entirely clear, beginning in 1943 the incidence of polio increased dramatically. In 1952 the polio rate reached 37.2 per 100,000 population, second only to 1916. That year saw over 57,000 contract the disease, the worst year in absolute numbers. In addition, as Dr. Dorothy Horstmann of the Yale Poliomyelitis Unit noted, between 1935 and 1955 there had been "a marked shift in the age distribution of the disease, with a steady decrease in the percentage of cases occurring in young children, and a continually increasing percentage in young adults." In addition, there was also evidence that "susceptible adults, when exposed, are more apt to develop severe infections with a high mortality."[19] For example, in the 1916 epidemic, about 80 percent of the cases occurred in children age four and younger. In 1949, slightly more than 20 percent of the cases were diagnosed in children age four and under, and 40 percent were in individuals older than ten.[20]

The fears of disease, crippling, and death in the polio years were real, but they were also enhanced by the poster child fund-raising campaigns of the March of Dimes, by the widespread cautions of the NFIP on how to avoid polio, by the media attention given to the dramatic accounts of any local epidemic, and by frequent closings of schools, swimming pools, movie houses, and other public gathering places when an epidemic loomed. The polio epidemics also threatened America's post–World War II longing to return to some kind of normalcy after fifteen years of depression and war. As one father put it, "Polio kills that. It stops that dream. It cuts it short."[21] The sociologist Fred Davis observed that "the child's contracting of the disease . . . loomed for the family as a kind of discriminatory barrier in the attainment of important social values; in short, it was 'un-American.'"[22] Thus the congruence of the worst decade in the history of polio in the United States with the well-oiled publicity machine of the NFIP and the cultural and social shift to the suburban good life made the disease something fearsome.

After a decade (1944–1955) in which over 361,000 cases of polio were diagnosed, the epidemics finally began to recede following the successful trial of the Salk vaccine in 1954 and the beginning of mass vaccination in 1955. Still, it took time for the Salk vaccine, supplemented by the Sabin vaccine after 1962, to eliminate epidemic polio.[23] Although the Salk vaccine made significant progress in ending the threat of polio in the United States, it was only with the widespread use of the Sabin oral vaccine that polio decreased to a relative handful per year.

Polio as an epidemic disease in the United States lasted barely seventy years, but in that time it became the most feared disease of childhood and adolescence. Those who lived through that time, whether as polio patients, anxious parents, overworked doctors and nurses, or March of Dimes volunteers will never forget the fear associated with polio and summers. Those fears, as well as the courage and determination to fight polio, are evident in the accounts that follow.

THE EARLY YEARS: 1916–1929

Pearl Piageri contracted polio in Corona, NY, in 1916 when she was eleven months old.

I was eleven months. We were quarantined to our house. There were so many of us that got polio at that time. It was a big epidemic. I went to a special school that was built for polio people. Some of us could walk into the bus. Some had to be carried on the bus, so there was a driver and an attendant. The school was handicap-accessible. We had treatment rooms where they would massage our legs and heat them up, and give us exercises, in addition to our regular classroom. The teachers were really good. We also had nurses that would come in. It was really a wonderful school.

Anthony DiBona contracted polio in New York City in 1916, forty days after his birth.

I contracted polio during one of the biggest epidemics in history—a thousand babies died that year in New York City alone. They used to tell the mothers to tickle the babies underneath their feet. If they would retract them, they were all right. My mother tickled my feet, the right one I withdrew and when she tickled my left one, I stood still.

There was a hospital on 42nd Street called Hospital for Crippled Children. I was in there for a couple of years. I was a breastfed baby. My mother used to have to come down twice a day to feed me—she would take the trolley car.

The 1930s

Bernice Lang contracted polio in Cleveland, OH, in 1930 when she was nine years old.

We were quarantined, and it was pretty rough. My older sister was in high school, but she wasn't allowed to go to school either. It was something for my mother to keep the four of us from fighting. She was worried that they shouldn't hurt me, and I shouldn't hurt them. They did their schoolwork because they had their schoolwork sent to them. They played games. There was no television then. There was radio. I don't think they were let out during the day, but at night my mother took them out for some air. My father was the only one of the family that was allowed to go outside because somebody has to make money. He went up to the school and told the teachers what had happened, and everybody was very cooperative, gave me books and papers to do at home. When I got done with them, my father took them back to school, and the teacher put them outside on the windowsill because she was afraid to let the other kids touch them.

Madeline Emerson's husband invented the iron lung.

My husband, John Haven Emerson, invented the iron lung. His was not the first iron lung. Philip Drinker in Boston, who was with Children's Hospital, had designed the first iron lung.... My husband invented the iron lung that was used during the polio epidemics.

Ironically, my husband developed polio himself. He had to go in the iron lung briefly. It left him with a partly paralyzed throat, so he couldn't eat well.

Polio began to be a real tragedy in the twenties, even more so in the thirties during the depression. We were told to stay out of swimming pools in the summer, and schools were closed.

My husband was in on the beginnings of the worry.

We'd go around the country to fundraising events. The March of Dimes grew out of that effort. We would go to these services groups and demonstrate the iron lung. These are the groups who bought them and donated them to hospitals. The way we sold our apparatus was, we had representatives around the country; we had about eight. They'd have a whole section of the country and they would demonstrate, sell and get a commission. We probably sold two or three hundred a year. We initially sold them for $2,000. The reps that we set up all around the country were in charge of servicing them.

Drinker sued my husband because he said that my husband took over what he had been trying to do. We went to court in Cambridge, and we had a very eminent lawyer. My husband was affiliated with the Harvard School of Public Health and Harvard was not supposed to allow apparatus that was invented there to be commercialized. But this was lifesaving equipment. This lawyer took the case because he felt my husband was helping people. When the case was finally closed in our favor, the lawyer didn't take a cent.

The 1940s

Frank McNally contracted polio in Southampton, NY, in 1947 when he was seven years old.

I was seven years old and Southampton was a very rural area. There was not very much polio out there. We were very much aware of polio because most of the newspapers that we read came out of New York City, and polio was a big story. There was always a concern that you might get it swimming. In eastern Long Island there were a lot of duck farms, and there was concern about, "Oh, you don't want to swim in the bays where those ducks are raised, you've got to swim in the ocean." I didn't have any restrictions, other than my parents said, "Go to the ocean."

After I had polio, there was a gal who was ahead of me in school came down with it, and she didn't walk away from it. She came out with the heavy braces and the Canadian crutches, but she did not let it get her down. She ended up being the queen of the senior prom. She went to work, and there was no assist for people that were challenged. She had stairs to climb, and she did it, and she really put a face on polio for my town. She was one of the most heroic people I ever met.

James Yamazaki, M.D., served in World War II and became a prisoner of war during the Battle of the Bulge. Following the war, he was a pediatric resident at Children's Hospital in Cincinnati, OH, from 1947–49.

In 1949, there was a large polio epidemic. One of the residents contracted polio. We were good friends, and he had already made plans to open his practice. He contracted polio while he was finishing his training and I was the chief resident. He immediately realized that he had developed bulbar polio and had to be in the iron lung. Because of the rapidity in which he developed symptoms, he asked me to give him morphine to put him away. He pleaded with me because he thought that if he survived it would be quite a tortuous path for him in the future. I told him I couldn't do that. He was still in the iron lung when I left the hospital. He eventually was removed from the iron lung and became professor of pediatrics at the University of Cincinnati. He was the only one of the residents that contracted the illness, and we were all exposed in a similar fashion.

Dr. Albert Sabin was the principal attending physician during the epidemic. Dr. Sabin was insistent that we kept very careful records, and he looked at the charts of each patient carefully. He was especially insistent that we provide the stool specimen according to his requirements. We followed his instructions. His principal interest was in the polio, and we knew that—When they were doing the oral polio initiative to try to get neighbors to take the sampling of the oral polio, he said that he had given it to his own daughters.

William Zanke contracted polio in Wheeling, WV, in 1949 or 1950 when he was four years old.

About six years ago, my brother and I went on vacation together, and he was telling me a story that when I had polio, they put up quarantine signs on the house. My two brothers were down the street. There was what we call a crick, C-R-E-E-K, and they were down by the waterside, and there's this big six-foot-tall sheriff standing at the top of the hill telling them they're not allowed out of the house, and they're both mildly intimidated. They noticed when they got to the top of the hill that the officer backed away from them so that they wouldn't get too close to him. It's only in later life that you realize the impact that your polio had on the rest of the family. It wasn't until I was a parent that I realized what it must have been like for my parents to have a kid with polio.

Mike Pierce, contracted polio in Southington, CT, in 1949 when he was five years old.

I was the first case reported in the town of Southington. The newspaper clipping that I was just given recently described that I was the first polio case in that town, and for the people not to worry because I had been removed.

There was a gentleman who raised a petition against my family. My mother and father lost all their friends. We were forced to move. My parents didn't tell me about this until later on. They told me about the man that started the petition to get us out of the neighborhood. I took care of that when I met this man. At first I thought I was going to kill him because of what he did to my folks. When I met him, I was a full-grown man. I stood up as tall as I could, and I was so much taller than this other guy. I took his hand in mine. I could have crushed it, and I just shook it. I said, "Pleased to meet you." When he looked at me, his eyes averted; I knew I won. He just shuffled away. He was beaten; he was whipped.

Katherine Pappas contracted polio in Cambridge, MA, in 1944 when she was five years old.

It was in August, around my birthday. We went swimming. A couple of days later, I couldn't walk. My mom thought that I was fooling, and I kept falling. I wasn't diagnosed until five days after that. Again, she thought I kept on either lying or I was just playing. I remember not being able to walk on my right leg.

We had a party that Saturday night because my cousin was going abroad in the service. We had a doctor attend this party. It was Governor Dukakis' father, and he was a doctor in Boston. He took one look at me and said, "Oh, my gosh, this is a sick gal." That was the end of the party, and I was rushed to Children's Hospital in Boston.

Ted Kellogg contracted polio in Westfield, MA, in 1943 when he was five years old.

The year that I got polio, there were two cases in Springfield: myself and a girl in the Indian Orchard section. She passed away. I was five and a half years old, and I went to Springfield Municipal Hospital. I remember being separated from my mother, me saying goodbye to her and her crying hysterically, "Don't say goodbye. That means I'll never see you again." I was there for about six weeks before they transferred me to the Newington Home for Crippled Children in Connecticut, where I stayed until I was eight or nine years old. They told my parents that they couldn't do anything more for me, and I went home for a year and a half before my parents were able to place me in the Massachusetts Hospital School in Canton, where I stayed until I was seventeen years old.

Irja Hoffshire was a physical therapist during the polio epidemics.
Before I became a physical therapist, I had the opportunity to work at a camp run by the Maryland League for Crippled Children at Camp Greentop. Now it is Camp David. Only severely handicapped children were allowed to come as campers. I was invited to become the assistant director of the girls' unit at Camp Greentop. I was there for 12 years. The children had come directly from the hospital after having suffered poliomyelitis. The camp was planned by President Roosevelt, FDR, because he had been a victim of poliomyelitis. He wanted children to have the opportunity to go to camp to make it feel like they were not handicapped. We had a swimming pool. The children loved it. They could do a lot more in the pool than they could do out of the pool. We had fifty girls and fifty boys. About 50% had polio.

President FDR did plan everything—the kind of housing for wheelchairs. Some of the campers had to lie on plinths. They couldn't sit up in a wheelchair. This was run by Secretary of Interior Harold Ickes.

The campers came from different walks of life. We had children from very wealthy homes. We had children from very deprived homes. The ones from deprived homes did not dwell on their limitations in their own homes, but were so happy to be at Camp Greentop. We had programs where they could participate. Singing was the best activity because polio did not affect their ability to sing. We had campfire once a week. We had cookouts. We had sleepovers.

I watched the physical therapist do her work. I really knew that's what I wanted to do. When World War II broke out, they needed physical therapists and were willing to train them. The army sent me to the University of Wisconsin Medical School, and there the farmers were the victims of polio.

When I left the army, I was married, and we decided to come to Massachusetts from Georgia. That was 1947. I applied immediately for a job as a physical therapist at our City Hospital. Poliomyelitis was very much in the active stage. I worked at the Belmont Hospital and in Worcester, which was for contagious diseases and polio patients. At City Hospital, I had a few polio patients, but not as many as at Belmont Hospital. When those patients were discharged, I would also go to their homes and do home therapy.

When I was working with patients who had polio, we had to be so careful. I had to scrub, before I went in, after I came out, change my shoes. I had two little children when I was working in Worcester, and my neighbor's children weren't allowed to play with my children until I convinced them that I was safer than the people they sat on the bus with because I took precautions. At Belmont hospital there were visiting hours. Parents couldn't come any time of the day they felt like coming because the children had to have their therapy. Therapy consisted of iron lungs and the hot packs and the exercise, whether they could move anything or not, and we had to do muscle testing.

Diana Barrett contracted polio in Mexico City in 1946 when she was one year old.

I didn't know anyone else who had polio, but I got to know a number of people in the next few years who had the disease—mostly Americans living in Mexico who didn't have any kind of protection against the disease. A significant number of Americans contracted polio at the time. After leaving the hospital I was brought to live in a high rise. There was such an incredible fear of coming down with polio. I was never allowed to be in the streets of Mexico. I was only allowed to be on the roof terrace. This is from the time I was born.

The rest of my childhood was going from one quack-like treatment to the next. When I was six or seven I went to a grueling and very painful series of cod liver injections into my leg. I remember being wrapped up like a mummy for weeks at a time and not being allowed to move. No one really knew what was going on, and the nature of the disease and the degree to which it affected nerves in your spinal column was still vague to people. My mother was searching for one treatment after another, and I don't remember any of them really having an effect until I actually had surgery when I was twelve, and that had a very clear, positive effect.

Lucille Hall contracted polio in Tennessee in 1946, sometime in the first year of life.

My mama was exposed to the virus when she was in her first trimester with me, and when I started walking, my mom noticed something wrong. She took me to the doctor, and that's what they told her. I was having trouble walking, and they kept me in the hospital for a while to see if physical therapy would work. I was only seventeen months old, so that was kind of young to really see if they could do anything.

THE 1950s

Jody Leigh Griffin contracted polio in Anchorage, AK, in 1954 when she was three years old.

I was the first case in Alaska in 1954. I was three years old. I never heard whether there was an epidemic that year. The doctors suspected that my sister had been exposed, and she had a mild case without any real symptoms. We didn't know anyone with polio. We were in Anchorage, and it was very sparsely populated.

Edward O'Connor contracted polio in the Bronx, NY, in 1955 when he was ten years old.

August 22, 1955. That was the date I was turned into the hospital. I used to go to the country, and it was towards the end of August. We'd been playing in a pond and fishing. The week prior to my commitment to the hospital was a Sunday. I was at church with my mother, and I started getting sick and nauseous. It was a very hot day, so someone had a smelling salt—they called it summer flu.

It was the following Friday. I was out with my older brother and friends. We had been swimming in the pond, and fishing, Huckleberry Finn type stuff, and we were walking home near supper because we were all hungry. I wasn't hungry that night, which was very rare for me, and I started feeling pain in my back and I started to limp on my right side. Not bad, but it was something I'd never experienced before. I started having a headache, so I went to bed because I didn't feel good.

During the night, I started getting a sore throat, headache, pain in my back. My mother called the doctor. He came into the house and he was talking to me. It was in the middle of the night—In those days anytime you had anything wrong, you had bowel trouble. "Do you need an enema?"

He came back the next day, and I was kind of feeling blah. I didn't want to get out of bed or anything, but no one told me what they suspected.

Saturday night it got real bad. I started getting nauseous, the throat started to close up. My mother called the doctor and he came. It was a Sunday, early morning, eight, nine o'clock. Then they were talking outside. Still didn't know what was going on.

The next thing I know, they put me in the ambulance. We were living in a town called Patchogue, Long Island, New York, and on the other side of Long Island is Port Jefferson, and there is a St. Charles Hospital that was built for polio. All over the hospital there was no stairs; it was all ramps. They transported me with the sirens going all the way across. That was quite an adventure.

Steven Diamond, M.D., contracted polio in the Bronx, NY, in 1953 when he was thirteen years old.

There was a Boy Scout camp that was closed because of an outbreak of polio at the camp. One of my friends was at that camp. My mother told me not to play with him, which, I did. Maybe shared an ice cream with him, and I came down with polio. I'm assuming he was the carrier; although, I can't prove this. When I was admitted to Bellevue Hospital, in the next bed to me was his bunkmate from the Boy Scout camp, who died.

I wound up at Bellevue Hospital for three and a half months. I remember an intern standing at the foot of my bed telling me I would never walk again. That was an impetus to walk. I remember telling him to go fuck himself, at age thirteen. That's when I decided to go into medicine.

I was in a wheelchair, kind of the big old wooden wheelchairs that Franklin D. Roosevelt was in. I would steal ice cream at night from this huge refrigerator and feed it to all the kids that were in the respirators. I have vague recollections of a Hubbard tank being put in there, a lot of hot packs. I walked out of there without leg braces or anything.

Most of my life has been spent in Bellevue Hospital. I'm a professor of medicine there, taught there, patient there. During my residency, I got called to the emergency room. I went down this corridor, and I had a panic attack. I wasn't somebody that ever had a panic attack, not even being shot at in Vietnam. Went back upstairs, came down again, the same thing happened. I put the lights on in the hallway, and it was the old rehab division in Bellevue. Everything came back to me. My mother used to take me there after I got out of the hospital. My name was carved in the wood bench. I remembered the names of all the people.

The next morning, I went down there, and I didn't even know that there was an old rehab unit still there. The physical therapist just about jumped all over me. She remembered me. I was thirteen, and now I was like twenty-eight. They threw a huge party for me. That was a very traumatic experience for me at that time.

Judith Willemy describes what it was like in Lowell, MA, in 1954.

In elementary school, we were told that we were going to see somebody who had polio. We weren't really quite sure what this is, but we knew it was a terrible thing. It was some terrible thing that happened to you if you didn't obey your parents, or if you didn't finish your meal, or if you fought with your brother and sister, or if you went swimming. Swimming was really the way to get polio, so you definitely could not go swimming.

We all lined up, and outside the school was a large truck. We went up the stairway in the front into this truck, and in the middle of the truck was a child laying on a table in a capsule, and the only thing showing was her head, and above her head was a mirror. You knew that this child had polio, which meant that she couldn't walk, but she was in this large capsule, so how much of her body was left?

We are wondering had she done that terrible thing, gone swimming? We just walked past her, gazing upon this scene, almost like at a sideshow in a circus. When we were children, we went to the circus and saw the little people, they were like dolls that were alive. We didn't know if they were really people. It was like that walking past this child. Is she real, and how much of her body is in that capsule? Oh my goodness, I hope this never happens to me. She'll spend the rest of her life in that capsule and never be able to come out, and how awful.

You really weren't sure if you had observed a human being or something that was almost like a sideshow. It just left a real impression of how we weren't taught that this was a person, how this person must have felt as children were going by. It was a terrible experience, and I'm really sorry that that child had to suffer that way.

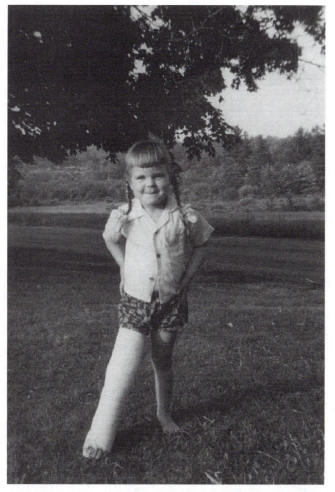

Ann Hussey, who was diagnosed with polio at seventeen months old, remembers she was living in Maine then, in 1955, and "it was back at the time when they used to put announcements in the newspapers: the daughter of Mr. and Mrs. Hussey has contracted polio." Photo courtesy of Ann Hussey.

Ann Lee Hussey contracted polio in North Berwick, ME, in 1955 when she was seventeen months old.

When I got polio it was back at the time when they used to put announcements in the newspapers: "the daughter of Mr. and Mrs. Hussey had contracted polio." With all the privacy acts, you don't get that these days.

The whole neighborhood pitched in. The neighborhood would take turns cooking dinners so that every evening, my mom didn't have to worry about when the next meal was coming.

Philip Thorpe contracted polio at William Field in Chandler, AZ, in 1952 when he was twenty-three years old.

I was in the Air Force. It was 1952, December 19th, the last day I walked like I used to. I was twenty-three. I was flying jets in the Air Force. I'd finished all the training and was waiting for graduation, which was going to be in three or four days. I went out of the barracks to my car. It had a flat tire, so I opened the trunk, tried to lift the spare out, and I was feeling like I had a virus. I had a backache, sort of hot, perspiring. I couldn't lift the spare tire out of the trunk. I thought, "Well, that's sort of weird," because I'm a big, strapping guy. I went back to the barracks and went to bed. A few hours later, I got up to go to the head, and I had to walk down two or three stairs. As I went down the stairs, my leg went out. There were lots of guys around, and I asked one of them to get my tactical officer. I said, "Lieutenant, I can't walk." He looked at me and felt my head. They took me to the base hospital in an ambulance and put me to bed.

There were two or three days when they had no idea what was wrong with me. I was sleeping. I had a fever, and I was in the hot stage of polio; although, it took at least three days for them to figure it out. They did that through a spinal tap. They did one, and they botched it—then did the second one, and they got the results from the Phoenix hospital.

They immediately put me into Phoenix Memorial in Arizona, which was a polio hospital. 1952 was one of the biggest epidemics of all time in the summer, and here it is the next winter. I'm one of the last to get it.

Earl P. "Chuck" Charlton contracted polio in California in 1954 when he was twenty-six years old.

When I got polio, I was assistant manager for the Woolworth Company. I went to the store in the morning and I was feeling very weak. My neck and arms ached, and I just wasn't feeling very well. I decided that I'd better see a doctor, but I didn't know what kind of doctor to go to, so I went to the pharmacist, and he asked me what symptoms I had. He says, "I think you ought to go to a doctor." He recommended Dr. Boggs, so I went to him. This doctor was very cognizant of polio and said, "I think we'd better get you in the hospital." I said, "I can't do that. I have a date this weekend." He said, "If you don't go to the hospital, we're going to send an ambulance after you."

I stayed in the hospital for about a month and a half. I would have stayed in the hospital longer, except the insurance company had refused to pay for any of the expenses, and I left early. I shouldn't have; I had a relapse, ended back up in the hospital.

Thelma Van Liew contracted polio in New Jersey in 1950 when she was six months old.

I remember hearing moans and groans of older people who were in the rooms next to us, and they were Caucasian, and we were on the other side—Edwina Jackson, myself, and a few other children who were Afro-American. We were separated from the elderly people, but they were still on the same floor. There wasn't a wall or anything. They were just down that end of the room, and we were down on this end. Back then nurses, doctors, interns seemed to care more for their patients in general, and it wasn't too much about the dollar like it is now. I got pretty good treatment. I wasn't dirty and nasty, and my parents didn't have to come and wash me up because they left me dirty all day and they couldn't get around to me.

Sylvia M. Barker was born in 1914 and became a nurse in 1933 at the age of nineteen. She was the nursing supervisor of pediatrics at the Mount Sinai Hospital in New York, NY, during the 1950s.

In the forties, when we had an epidemic of acute polio, we had a visit from Sister Kenny from Australia. She came and demonstrated her system of treating polio with the hot packs, which we used on our pediatric units. We had no air conditioning. To use hot, steamy packs on a hot, steamy day was very trying. We had to run those hot packs through those wringers and then wrap them up in a waterproof covering so that the bed wouldn't get too wet. It did help the children to relieve some of their discomfort, and they were able to get some sleep.

I wasn't concerned about contracting polio. As a nurse, we were taught what we were supposed to do in terms of washing our hands, keeping things clean about us, and our direct contacts with the patients, so that we would not contract a disease or transmit it.

In 1953 we opened the Jack Martin Polio Respirator Center in my department. The unique thing about that Respirator Center was that it was open to adults and children who were impaired as far as their respirations were concerned. In the fifties most units were segregated; males and females, children and adults. Our hospital was not racially segregated. Mount Sinai is a Jewish hospital, and that's one thing that's just not done. We opened it first in September 1953, and the first unit that we created were temporary quarters, which had the capacity of about seven patients. Then in November 1955, we moved into the renovated area that became the Jack Martin Polio Respirator Center.

The unit was dedicated on January 6, 1959. One of the persons present at the dedication was the actress Helen Hayes, who had become very interested in rehabilitation matters. She dedicated the plaque in memory of Jack Martin. He was a thirty-four year old man who developed polio and died after a very brief encounter with the disease. He was a manufacturer in the garment industry, and after he died, his sister led a group of two hundred women who wanted to perpetuate his memory. They raised funds and came in contact with the National Polio Foundation when the foundation was beginning to think about the development of these Respirator Centers. Ours at Sinai was one of twelve centers that were developed across the Unites States. Ours was the eighth. These centers flourished up until the development of the Salk vaccine. After the Salk vaccine came polio disappeared, and the centers were no longer needed. Ours closed on June 15, 1960.

The last patient was transferred on June 15, 1960. She went to her home. Four patients died while in our care; three were established in apartments with attendants; one was transferred to Goldwater; and two became free from need of respiratory aid and were transferred to general rehab units. That gives some idea of the distribution of the patients and the outcome of the care that they received. The three common types of respiratory assistive devices that we were using were the typical tank-type respirator, which is sometimes known as the "Drinker" respirator, chest respirators, and a rocking bed.

In addition to these respiratory assistive devices, the patients needed good nursing care, physical therapy, occupational therapy, psychiatric assistance, and social workers. There were nurses' aides who were helpful to the professional nurses in giving care, moving patients, lifting patients. These patients could not move on their own. We had a group of workers on the unit called ward helpers. They were the ladies that helped with serving food and keeping the place clean. We had male orderlies to assist with the care of male patients. The adult patients in the unit were usually fairly young. They were women in their reproductive years. They were men in their twenties and thirties. I don't believe we had too many people beyond forty in the unit. One of the things of great concern to these patients was their sexual life to follow this catastrophic event, so this was training that we tried to provide; help them understand how they could become effective sexual partners following their return home. It was done through group teaching and the experience that the psychiatrists and other physical therapists were able to share with the patients.

When I was a student nurse, a child came into the hospital and he or she did not see his parents again for two weeks. I thought that was perfectly horrible, and so as soon as I became supervisor, I began to make a change. Ultimately, we have very liberal visiting hours for children in most hospitals, and in the Respirator Center we did have very liberal visiting hours. We allowed visitors to come in the morning, the afternoon, or the evening, whichever was convenient for the relative. In the Respirator Center we allowed children and infants to come and visit. These women had children at home they wanted to see. In the notes that I was reviewing for this interview, I found a little note that said, "There even was small animals that managed to get in during visiting hours."

I asked the nurses' aides to keep a little diary for a two-week period of what they did for the patients. I was trying to see if their functioning on the unit was profitable and what type of thing they did. I expected to find entries such as feeding the patients or turning the patients or helping the nurse to get the patient out of bed. I found an entry, which said, "Smoked the patient." Our patients were allowed to have a cigarette. Because they were paralyzed, they couldn't hold it, so the nurses' aide would hold the cigarette for the patient to smoke. The nurses' aide had dubbed this "Smoked the patient." This gives a little idea about making the care that we gave the patient as compassionate as possible. With all the emphasis today on not smoking, we wouldn't have encouraged that kind of thing, but in those days, smoking was very common. We also encouraged giving of permanent waves, because the female patients needed to have their hair taken care of.

William Berenberg, M.D., was a pediatrician at Children's Hospital in Boston, MA, during the 1955 polio epidemic.

The hysteria in the city was beyond description. Anybody who had a kid that was not feeling well, in the minds of the parents, they had polio until proven otherwise. They used to come running to the hospital to be evaluated. They had their own doctor see them. Very often the doctor would say there's no need to come, you don't have it. Or he might say I'm not sure. You need a spinal tap to find out. And would send them in, then they would get their tap right then and there, if it was indicated. There was a tremendous influx of people. On the busiest nights we'd get deluged because a lot of people did not have automobiles. They used to wait till daddy got home with the car. Then they'd pile in and go to the hospital. If you had 150 or 200 of them hit you at about the same time, it was bad. The police held them in an orderly line. They could not leave their spot in line to be examined and beat the wait unless they had a red card. Dr. Grice and I, David Grice, who was an orthopedist, used to do a lot of our preliminary screening in the automobile. Each of us had large-size floodlights and we'd look in the car. If the kid was playing, looked mobile, he stayed in line. The ones who were obviously in either respiratory distress or couldn't move an arm, we would give a card to so they could go up to the head of the line. The worst night was that line went back to the Meeting House of Temple Israel on the Riverway. Lined solid with automobiles full of children. It's more than a half a mile. We spent the whole night just going back and forth.

Jonathan Salk, M.D., is the youngest child of Jonas Salk (he had three sons).

My dad was a very warm and physically present father. Throughout his life, his main involvement was his work. Family was important to him, and he didn't disregard it, but when push came to shove, what was on his mind were the work priorities and the important things. In the years before the vaccine— the success of the vaccine was announced when I was almost five—he worked long hours, and he traveled to conferences, but he was around a fair amount.

The years following the vaccine really did change his life. He had many more responsibilities. He was very preoccupied with a lot more complicated things. As a child, I was completely aware of polio. We visited the Watson Home for crippled children outside Pittsburgh, and those were the children who were the first human beings who received the polio vaccine in some preclinical trials. I did not have any sort of personal fear of the disease. Fear was prevalent everywhere, but it was never something that I lived with.

After the vaccine, we went down to Warm Springs, Georgia. I remember very vividly seeing the different kinds of apparatuses that crippled children had to wear and use, and page-turners, and rolling drums to help them breathe.

My dad was on the cover of Time magazine, and we had a picture of him sur-rounded by syringes and needles, and braces and crutches. Our lives changed after the announcement of the polio vaccine. We went to Ann Arbor for the announcement of the vaccine. We were going to be there overnight and come back. Nobody had any idea what a huge news story it was going to be. We literally couldn't leave Ann Arbor for several days because there was so much going on. When we got back to Pittsburgh there was a reception at the airport, and a motorcycle escort back to our house.

There was the Cutter incident, where some children got polio from a bad batch of the vaccine. I remember that being really troubling to my dad. Fol-lowing the announcement was actually a distressing time for my father. He felt that what he had done and what the vaccine did was not accepted by the scientific community because of the whole controversy between the killed vaccine and the live virus vaccine. He was really distressed and sort of not knowing what to do because there was all this acclaim, but everybody was regarding this as a stopgap measure.

From my father's point of view, I don't believe that he felt or saw a personal rivalry with Albert Sabin. He felt that Sabin did feel that way. They were completely different personalities. I've heard from many people that Albert Sabin was a bombastic, kind of intellectually aggressive, somewhat vitupera-tive guy, and he rubbed a lot of people the wrong way. My father tended to be sort of quiet, gracious, avoid conflict; although, he certainly had his share of conflict. In terms of the rivalry between them, on a public health level was the question as to which vaccine was more effective. My father always felt that the killed virus vaccine by itself had the capacity to contain polio. What he felt and worked very hard at, was that once wild virus polio was not around, in the United States, there were a small number of five or six vaccine-associated cases associated with the live virus vaccine. My father always felt that it was an unacceptable risk that since there was an effective vaccine that didn't cause the disease, there wasn't any reason to do that. The decision to go with the live vac-cine in the early sixties was something that was distressing and painful to him.

As far as the personal rivalry between them, my dad didn't talk about it very much. I was aware that periodically Sabin would say disparaging things about my father, in terms of what my father had done and the nature of the work that he did. It wasn't experienced in my family as a personal competition and that my dad was racing with Sabin to make a successful vaccine. My father was just focused on getting a vaccine done, and getting it out to help people as quickly as possible.

THE 1960s AND AFTER

Justine Guckin contracted polio in Newington, CT, in 1969 when she was two years old.

I was two years old when I contracted polio from the live vaccine. It wasn't my vaccine, though. I had gotten it from another person in my neighborhood who had gotten the live vaccine. Somehow we exchanged, whether it was spit on a toy or whatever—we were two—so any kind of bodily fluids passed through. When I was supposed to get the third vaccine, I did not because I had a bad ear infection. My immune system was low, and when I came in contact with the other person who got vaccinated with the live vaccine I contracted it. It was around Memorial Day, and I was walking in the yard. I was fine up until this point, and I fell in the yard, and I couldn't get up. I was crying, and my mother brought me to the doctor's. The doctor didn't know what it was, and they put me into St. Raphael's Hospital. It was a long time before they figured it out because they couldn't believe that in 1969 this could be polio. I was the first one in years to catch it where I lived. They had to rule out everything else before they finally pinpointed that it was polio.

2

ACUTE AND CONVALESCENT POLIO

In an era when family physicians still made house calls, polio was usually diagnosed at home. Sometime in the late summer, a child, a teenager, or even a parent began to feel ill and soon developed a fever. If the fever persisted and was accompanied by nausea, increasing muscle pain, and a headache, the doctor was often called. But physicians didn't always initially diagnose the ailment as poliomyelitis. These were fairly common symptoms and polio was often difficult to diagnose correctly. No doctor wanted to make the wrong diagnosis. Once paralysis set in, the physician came again and pronounced the dreaded diagnosis in hushed, worried tones.[1] The ailing family member was soon hustled into the family car and quickly driven to the nearest hospital admitting acute polio patients.

The ride to the hospital was usually frightening. Bumpy roads and highways produced considerable pain in increasingly sensitive muscles. Most children had never been hospitalized previously, and some had never been away from home. Even very young children could sense the fear and anxiety in their parents' eyes and behavior. During polio epidemics particular hospitals were often designated to admit and treat these patients. This often meant a drive of many miles to reach the nearest hospital handling polio patients. African American families in this era of segregation often had to find the nearest black hospital, or travel considerable distance to find a segregated hospital that would admit their child.[2] Dr. Thomas Daniel, who treated polio patients at Haynes Hospital in Boston during the 1954 epidemic, observed, "Polio was a dreaded disease, even among doctors, and these terrified, sick people were immediately made to feel like pariahs, cast out to the Haynes Hospital."[3]

Several distinct memories of the arrival at the polio hospital stand out in the recollections of polio survivors. Although many incoming polio patients had been tentatively diagnosed, doctors frequently wanted to do a spinal tap to confirm the diagnosis. In this procedure the patient was lying on her side curled into a fetal position, and the doctor inserted a long needle into the

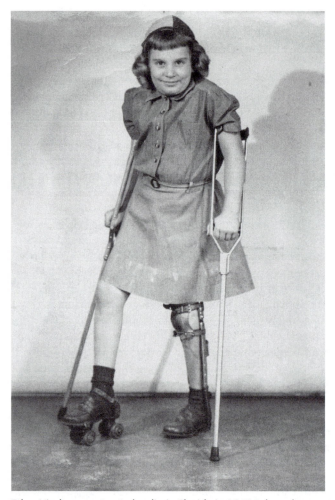

Edna Hindson contracted polio in Florida in 1946, when she was
six years old. Photo courtesy of Edna Hindson.

spine. He then extracted a small amount of fluid surrounding the spinal cord.
Certain changes to the cerebrospinal fluid were characteristic of polio. This
procedure was often quite painful and could produce excruciating headaches.
Patients were often not informed of the details of this procedure prior to un-
dergoing it. For children especially, the recollection of this procedure remains
a particularly horrific memory.[4] The other painful memory of this time was the
separation from parents or spouses. Sometimes good-byes were not possible
as patients were rushed directly to the ward. Other times, hurried good-byes
in the hallway were little consolation to new patients when the doors to the
isolation unit closed behind them. Most polio hospitals did not permit visitors
on the wards or in the rooms. Parents and spouses haunted waiting rooms

perhaps viewing their loved one through glass doors, or stood outside hoping for a glimpse through the window. Gowned and masked parents and spouses were sometimes admitted if physicians thought the patient was in danger of dying.

Many hospitals restricted visitors in order to reduce the chance of spreading the disease and to better manage their patients. Other hospitals, however, discovered that family members could relieve overburdened hospital personnel by helping to feed and care for their sons or daughters, husbands or wives.[5] In addition, by the 1950s polio scientists had come to realize that "by the time a physician is called to see a case, virtually all other susceptible members of the family have been infected, whether or not they have symptoms."[6] This explains why few of the parents and spouses who were allowed to visit and why relatively few of the medical and hospital personnel who cared for these patients contracted polio in spite of their hands on care.

Acute poliomyelitis could be quite painful depending on how extensively the virus had destroyed or damaged the nerve cells. Many patients had a high temperature and were nauseated. Some polio patients experienced searing muscle spasms and unaffected muscles could twist limbs and torsos into uncomfortable positions. Patients were also very sensitive to touch. And, if the virus attacked the nerves that controlled the muscles of respiration, polio patients could quickly find themselves struggling to breathe. Once the disease began, doctors had no way of altering its course. The most they could do was to try to make the patients comfortable for the week or more of the acute stage. Before the widespread adoption of Sister Kenny's methods, physicians recommended absolute rest, using frames to keep sheets off tender muscles, and placing limbs in casts to maintain normal positioning. Heat was also sometimes recommended, but drugs were seldom used except to relieve pain.[7] The gradual acceptance after 1940 of Sister Kenny's methods of using hot packs to reduce muscle spasm and pain significantly improved acute polio care. However, her methods still did nothing to alter the course of the disease.[8] The most memorable aspect of acute polio care in the forties and fifties was the application of these wet wool hot packs several times a day. With a flexible body, nurses and therapists could begin to reeducate muscles to their normal function as the disease receded.[9] While polio patients often welcomed the hot packs for the relief they provided, they also feared being burned by carelessly applied packs. And because polio was typically a summer disease, these hot packs were often endured during the sultry months in hospitals without air-conditioning.

One of the most frightening and dramatic moments of acute polio came when the advancing paralysis reached the muscles that controlled respiration and the patient began to struggle to breathe. Before Philip Drinker's invention of the iron lung in 1928 physicians could not save these patients. There are horrific accounts of how these patients would gasp for air and choke on their own secretions. The experimental success of the iron lungs and their commercial production and sale in the thirties and forties finally gave doctors a means of keeping patients with respiratory failure alive in the hope that they would regain sufficient muscle strength to be able to breathe on their own once again. Although they saved many lives, iron lungs posed challenges for physicians, nurses, and patients. Physicians initially worried that placing patients in the devices doomed them to a life entombed in the tank. Moreover, since only the sickest patients used the iron lungs, many still did not survive. Hence the nickname the "iron coffin." But as doctors and nurses became more accustomed to using the respirators a significant percentage of patients eventually recovered sufficiently to leave the iron lungs permanently.

In general, patients with spinal polio affecting the breathing muscles were more likely to survive than those who had bulbar polio, which also affected the swallowing muscles. The distinctions between spinal and bulbar polio were not always clear, and in such circumstance the doctors usually put the patient in the respirator. In severe epidemics doctors were sometimes forced to make agonizing choices when they had more patients needing assistance than they had iron lungs. In the early 1940s the National Foundation for Infantile Paralysis (NFIP) began to purchase iron lungs and to store them so that they could be quickly sent to communities needing them. That reduced the shortages of iron lungs, but doctors still agonized about possibly condemning patients to a lifetime dependence on them. However, as David Rothman observed, "confronting a dying patient, doctors would do something, anything, rather than just stand there, or even give comfort." Physicians came to feel that placing patients in the respirator was a risk worth taking.[10]

Fear of iron lungs was widespread because so many patients died in them and because the March of Dimes so successfully used the specter of the iron lung to raise funds. Many polio survivors recall the fear they felt on seeing their first iron lung or hearing the characteristic whoosh-whoosh of a working respirator. However, if they began to struggle for each breath, the large machines quickly lost their threatening aspect. Because paralysis of the breathing muscles could happen quickly, and because doctors, reluctant to place anyone in the respirator, sometimes waited too long, patients were often in considerable distress before being slid into the tank. Once the opening snapped shut and the bellows began to move air in and out of the patient's lungs, they felt immediate relief. They could breathe again and without a struggle. But with relief there was a new adjustment. One had to breathe according to the machine's dictates; the rate of respiration was determined by the doctor who adjusted the machine. Patients quickly discovered they could talk only when the machine expelled air from their lungs and conversations became disjointed. Many also discovered that they were completely paralyzed and unable to move a muscle voluntarily. They couldn't scratch an itch, move to a more comfortable position, cover or uncover themselves, feed themselves, or take a drink of water. They were totally dependent on someone else to do all the ordinary things they had done only hours or days earlier. Caring for patients in iron lungs was difficult for the medical and nursing staff. To care for these patients, nurses had to reach through portholes in the side of the tanks. Opening a porthole reduced the pressure in the lung and patients struggled to breathe, so speed was essential. Caring for patients in iron lungs was "constant and relentless."[11]

The acute phase of poliomyelitis came to an end when the spread of paralysis ended and the patient's fever subsided. This might be a week to ten days after onset. Many of these patients remained seriously ill. They were still weak from their ordeal, and most continued to have muscular paralysis. However, they began to be more aware of their circumstances and began to assess the damage the disease had done. At this point, most were moved out of the isolation ward to a convalescent ward. This move to a polio ward was a significant step. They were feeling better and could interact with their ward mates. Nurses and doctors were not gowned and masked, which made them less threatening. There were normal visiting hours, which if still too short, nonetheless allowed contact with family. Most still faced weeks, perhaps months of hospitalization, but this was clearly the first important step to returning home.

Convalescence from polio was a long-term project and usually involved intensive rehabilitation efforts. Most physicians believed convalescence began forty-eight hours after the patient's fever ended and continued until "no further recovery in musculature is to be expected." The end point generally occurred sixteen to twenty-four months following the onset of the disease.[12] When first moved to a convalescent ward, many polio patients were still suffering from painful muscle spasms and contractures and were very sensitive to touch. Dr. William Green argued that "the primary considerations in the early convalescent stage . . . are to make the patient comfortable, to avoid or at least minimize deformity, to develop increasing arcs of motion in the affected areas, and shortly thereafter to start active exercises for the paretic [paralyzed] muscles, all dominated by the importance of rest, both general and local."[13] During this early stage of convalescence doctors also tested and graded muscle function. Muscle grading was repeated throughout the recovery and gave physicians and polio survivors a means of gauging progress.

Once the patient's sensitivity disappeared, he or she was ready to begin a more sustained rehabilitation. The hot packs were typically discontinued at this point. Patients were encouraged to begin active exercises to strengthen weak muscles. The exercise regimen was individualized and designed to meet the particular needs of the patient. Some facilities contained warm pools where the buoyancy of the water made it easier to move weak or partially paralyzed limbs. Depending on the severity of the paralysis and the muscles affected, therapists eventually worked on enabling the patients to sit, stand, and walk. Doctors were reluctant to prescribe braces or other assistive devices initially in the hope that exercise would make such appliances unnecessary. The length of this in-hospital rehabilitation varied considerably. In a 1947 study of polio patients, 40 percent stayed for three weeks or less, 8 percent were hospitalized for at least six months, and 4 percent remained for a year or more. As Dr. William Green noted, "treatment is as simple and short or as long and detailed as necessary."[14]

The locations where recovering polio patients received therapy varied considerably. Some were treated at home with a visiting therapist or outpatient clinics providing parents with guidance in directing their child's exercises. In some cases, the rehabilitation wards were simply another part of the facility where they had suffered through acute polio. But many polio survivors experienced all or part of their rehabilitation in one of the numerous public or private rehabilitation hospitals. Many states and some counties and cities had public residential facilities for crippled children. These included Rancho Los Amigos in Downey, California, Gillette Children's Hospital in St. Paul, Minnesota, and the New York State Reconstruction Home in West Haverstraw, New York. Polio patients made up the bulk of the children treated for physical impairments from 1916 to 1960. Charitable organizations, such as the Shriners, also operated rehabilitation hospitals that served needy polio patients. Sister Kenny and her foundation also opened several facilities that treated patients according to her methods. And, finally, there was the Georgia Warm Springs Foundation. Many of the state and county hospitals were grim places with inadequate staffing, run-down facilities, and a minimum of appropriate therapy. However, other public institutions, such as Rancho Los Amigos, had an excellent reputation for polio rehabilitation. Among polio patients Warm Springs stood out, in part because of its association with Roosevelt, but also because it retained, in the estimation of those treated there, something of the feeling of its resort origins. Once the NFIP began paying for treatment and began setting standards, conditions and treatment improved somewhat, but there was still tremendous variation.

It was difficult for individual hospitals to care for long-term iron lung survivors and to wean them from the respirators. By moving these patients out of more than 135 hospitals to fifteen respiratory centers the NFIP promoted "research into how best to manage respirator therapy, acute and chronic," administered "training programs . . . for medical personnel," and provided better care for "the most difficult chronic cases." The National Foundation did not succeed in moving all respirator patients into one of its centers. However, a high percentage of patients treated at these centers eventually went home, many able to use smaller, more portable devices.[15]

Polio patients had mixed emotions on moving to a rehabilitation facility. It was, of course, a real sign of progress. Still, it often meant a long separation from family and friends. It was often difficult for family and friends to visit. However, new polio patients were quickly initiated into a flourishing ward culture. Because hospital stays were so long in this period, friendships quickly developed. They encouraged one another to persist with their therapy and exercises. They shared memories of the past and dreams for the future. If they were school age, they attended classes. There were jokes to tell, pranks to play, radios to listen to, and occasionally televisions to watch. They eagerly anticipated visits, and dreaded the loneliness in between. Once they became mobile, whether on braces and crutches or in wheelchairs, there were hospital corridors to explore.

One of the most challenging aspects of rehabilitation was weaning iron lung patients from their dependence on the device. As soon as the acute disease ended, doctors, nurses, and patients began the painful process. Typically, iron lung patients would be slid out of the lung for brief periods to see how long they could breathe. If they had any capacity to breathe on their own, the time out of the tank was increased slightly each day. These exercises were terrifying for patients dependent upon the iron lung, but they were also necessary. Some iron lung patients also learned to frog breathe (glossopharyngeal breathing) in which the neck muscles were used to force air into the lungs. As part of their transition out of the lung, some patients were moved to rocking beds whose motion provided some breathing assistance. In spite of the incessant rocking, patients generally liked the move as it got them out of the tank, made their care much easier, allowed them to see more of the world around them, and represented progress. Other respiratory patients were able to use cuirass or chest respirators that fit tightly around the chest. These allowed patients to sit up and, with more portable units, to use wheelchairs. A significant percentage of iron lung patients with spinal polio were eventually able to leave the iron lung either completely or for long periods, although some remained dependent on some type of respiratory assistance.[16]

Although the initial rehabilitation usually came to an end within two years of the onset of polio, being discharged from the rehabilitation hospital did not necessarily mean the end of therapy. Many polio survivors continued outpatient treatments. This might continue for several years until physicians, or in some cases the polio survivor, decided that little additional benefit was likely. When exercise did not restore function, many doctors recommended surgery to fuse joints or spines, or to transplant muscles and tendons to improve function. Generally these surgeries, often experimental, came several years after polio. With children and teenagers, doctors often recommended waiting with surgery until growth had slowed or stopped.[17] This meant that many polio survivors experienced one or more surgeries several years after they had finished physical therapy.

However extended, physical therapy and surgery eventually ended. Inevitably, at some point medicine could do no more to restore function and doctors discharged their patients. In some cases, polio survivors or their parents decided to end therapy or refused yet another surgery. They were satisfied with the level of functioning they had achieved, or simply gave up on the idea that further recovery was possible. Others wanted to put polio behind them and finish their education, get back to work, or care for their families. Doctors sometimes implied, if they did not explicitly promise, that the polio survivor's level of impairment would remain stable. Polio survivors had the consolation that it wouldn't get worse. Because post-polio syndrome would not be fully described until the 1980s, no one was warned of the potential for further problems that might appear decades later. Finally, the long painful journey through acute and convalescent polio came to an end. In spite of the fact that many polio survivors still relied on medical technology to help them sit, stand, walk, or breathe, they could now resume the life interrupted by their encounter with this terrible virus.

THE EARLY YEARS

Ruth Esau contracted polio in Cass City, MI, in 1919 when she was two years old.

On a Sunday morning in August, I awakened very cross and uncomfortable. We had been invited to go visit cousins in another town. I could still walk, but I wasn't well. My parents didn't think I was sick enough to stay home. When we got there, I couldn't walk. I fell down every time I tried to step. I played a little bit, but then my parents took me to see a doctor. This doctor knew immediately that it was beyond his ability to care for me. My mother just cared for me.

Then my brother came home sick. My father wasn't feeling well either, and his appendix burst. It all happened within six weeks. My brother got better, but my father died in the hospital in a coma within three days.

After my father died, I was taken in my mother's arms to Detroit, where she went from doctor to doctor. A doctor said to her, "The nerve feeding her left leg is not working." Eventually my mother settled with the leading orthopedic surgeon in Michigan; he was my doctor until I was fourteen.

My mother always had a little dish on this warm range with a bar of cocoa butter in it, and every night, she thoroughly massaged my left leg.

I was seven when my first surgery was done. Cords were cut, and I was put in a cast. Surgery was quite traumatic in those days. There was no discussion with me what was going to be done. I just knew I was going to be in the hospital for quite a while. I was whisked away down elevators and halls into the basement of the old Grace Hospital in Detroit and held forcibly on the table. I kicked and kicked. Finally, the ether was clamped over my nose, mouth, and I thought I was being killed. I woke up in a recovery room with a very kind doctor and my mother. Then I was put into the children's ward.

I stayed there a number of weeks. There were rows of children. I have the hard memory that the little girl next to me died. I had daily treatment of the wound. There was absolutely nothing like physical therapy.

After my second operation, I had to have specially-made leather shoes with a lift on the sole and the heel because my leg was shorter. I had to wear an iron brace that went from my hip. It was fastened to the shoe. It had a hinge at the knee that I could unlock when I sat down. Mom bought my shoes. They were thirteen dollars, which was a lot of money because she only made a dollar a day.

My family was wonderful. I loved school. My mom bought a little wicker stroller and pushed me in that to kindergarten. My brother took me in a little Express wagon or on a sled or on his bicycle. I had cousins that were in high school who would stop with a little pickup and give me a ride. I never could walk to school, and I had to take my lunch. The town children all walked home, but I had to stay with the country children.

When I came home, the big bed from upstairs had been placed in the living room, and for a long time, my mother and I slept downstairs because I couldn't go up.

THE 1930s

Alice Cote contracted polio in Attleboro, MA, in 1935 when she was twenty-two months old.

I had polio when I was twenty-two months old, but I wasn't hospitalized until I was three. My parents couldn't decide on my treatment. One of them believed in the chiropractor; the other one wanted me to have medical treatment. They were trying both methods. There was no improvement with my condition, so my parents signed papers to allow me to go to Lakeville Hospital with the understanding that they could not take me from there until the doctors released me. My mother died in 1939; I was six years old. I remember my father standing at the foot of the bed trying to tell me that my mother died. He tried to take me out so that I could go to the funeral. They wouldn't let me go. I think a lot of my surgeries were experimental. I was in the hospital until 1944. I was twelve when I came out.

I didn't know anyplace else—only the hospital. I was treated very rigidly. One time I was punished for something that I didn't even understand until I was in my forties. I had my head flushed down the toilet. That haunted me for a long time. I had some glue in my crib. I put it all over me. I was pretending to wash my hair. I remember the nurse finding me like that. She said the only way she was ever going to get all that out of my hair was to put my head down the toilet and flush it. When my kids were growing up I didn't even allow glue in my house, and I never could understand why. I used to always ask myself, "Why?" I would make flour and water paste. I finally discovered that it was this episode in the hospital.

Another time that I was punished was when I wouldn't drink tomato juice. I loved tomato juice. One day, I couldn't drink it because it smelled like a cellar. I was told, "Well, we'll show you what cellar is." They took the wheelchair and me, put me down in the cellar, and left me there for the whole day. I couldn't go into a cellar in my own home. It happened on a Sunday, the one visiting day. They wouldn't let me up out of the cellar for my company. That always bothered my father; he wanted to take me out of that hospital, but he couldn't.

THE 1940s

J. Phillip Kistler contracted polio while on vacation in La Jolla, CA, in 1943 when he was five years old.

Sister Kenny came to see me in the quarantine area in the hospital. I remember being loaded onto a stretcher, then taken by ambulance to the airport, and loaded on one of those DC-3s, with only a couple of seats in it. I was on the stretcher, strapped down, Sister Kenny was in a seat, and there was a nurse there. We flew off to Minneapolis. It was during the war, and pretty hard to get around in those days, particularly by air.

I stayed at the Sister Kenny Institute about three and a half months. We had a bunch of beds in the room, and a big area—those who could walk could play. I was in a bed with a bunch of bedrails. I was flat down.

Sister Kenny was involved in my daily care. You had a hot-pack team, and a team of stretchers who would stretch you, and physical therapy. They put the hot packs on you in your bed. They'd stretch you in your bed. They'd roll you down to the exercise area, and she had a big auditorium where she would demonstrate.

Margo Vickery contracted polio in New Jersey in 1946 when she was five years old.

Sister Kenny worked with polio patients and had a different system for caring for them. My mother went to hear her talk. The therapy for polio was keeping people in iron lungs, keeping them still. Sister Kenny would put warm cloths on the limbs that were affected, and have someone exercise the paralyzed arms and legs.

When I contracted polio I had a temperature of 106 for ten days. The doctors said that if I survived, I would be crazy, I would lose all my hair. None of those things happened. The doctors wanted me to go to the hospital. My father said, "Are you going to make her well?" They said, "No, we can't do that."

"Well, what are you going to do for her?"

"Well, we're going to put her in an iron lung and test things."

My father said, "No, you're not. My wife will take care of her."

That's why I didn't go to the hospital.

My mother took care of me. She remembered what Sister Kenny had taught her and she would carry me into the bathtub, take me back to bed, and physically make my limbs move. It hurt her and it hurt me, but I couldn't cry.

My mother was filled with fear and obligation and thought, "What am I going to do? How am I going to help my daughter?"

I often said to her, particularly before she died, "You know, you gave birth to me twice, once when I was born and the other when you saved me from dying from polio."

Bill Schweid, M.D., contracted polio in Okinawa, Japan, in 1947 when he was twenty-five years old.

I was stationed as a medical officer in Okinawa, Japan, in 1947 when I contracted polio. I had a severe headache. I took my temperature and it was at 103.0° Fahrenheit. I was a little nauseated. I was taken to our hospital, which was a Quonset hut with twenty patients in it.

They took a chest x-ray and it was perfectly normal. My only complaint was this headache and nausea. I developed severe pain in both calves, but it was relieved with aspirin. I didn't need anything more potent than that.

The next day, I had trouble getting to the washroom, but the captain who was in charge of the hospital insisted I walk. I dragged myself to the latrine. I was in a room with ten other men. I couldn't prop myself up with my left arm because I was so weak. The next day I couldn't move my left lower extremity . . . put me in a private room, which looked like a small cell in jail. They quarantined me.

My treatment was "Do not move." I didn't move. They did several lumbar punctures, and sent them to Washington, D.C. They also treated me with hypertonic plasma, which is double thick plasma powder diluted in saline solution. It was their theory that they were going to do something to my nerves to relieve swelling.

When I got back to the United States, I read the nurses' notes: "Patient constantly complaining. Insists on being fed. Urinated in a drinking glass." I had no other alternatives, and I insisted on being fed because I couldn't prop myself up on my left arm to feed myself.

I was medically discharged in June of 1948, one year later, and I was told to carry on with my life.

Mike Pierce contracted polio in Southington, CT, in 1949 when he was five years old.

The rough time was in the hospital. I don't remember whether I could move my arms. I couldn't move my legs, but I could move my head from side to side. Every single kid in there was crying.

We were allowed to listen to radio in the afternoon, if we ate our supper. One day I didn't eat my green beans. I was put out into the hall to listen to the radio with the others and this one nurse picked me up, said, "You didn't eat your green beans, so you don't get to listen to the radio." I was thrown back to bed. I cried and cried. I wanted to get out of there. I hated hospitals.

Katherine Pappas contracted polio in Cambridge, MA, in 1944 when she was five years old.

I remember being in this large ward, and my parents could only visit me on Saturday afternoon from two to four because they thought that parents would be disruptive. My priest came to visit me three times a week. I had a lot of faith. I was never frightened because I always had God with me.

I was in the hospital for two years. My dad owned a little grocery store so, he could never come to visit me. Saturday was a busy day, unfortunately. I remember Christmas, best Christmases I ever had because I got lots of gifts from people. My parents were very poor, so we just got oranges and apples in stockings. When I was in the hospital, I got fancy toys.

I had surgery. It felt like it was every summer. My surgeries absolutely helped me walk. I'd be in braces today if I didn't have them. I've had, over my lifetime, twenty-three surgeries.

The surgeries weren't traumatic for me because I was very comfortable in the hospital. I welcomed surgery. Even today, I welcome surgery.

I liked the hospital because there I was someone very special. In the Greek home, girls were not considered equal to boys. I had to do more housework, with braces and all. My mom went to work after I got polio. When I was ten years old, I had to start dinner. I couldn't play outside with the kids in the neighborhood because I had my chores to do. I resented that. Then I went to this very lovely Boston Children's Hospital, where I was treated like a queen.

My mom was devastated that something would happen to her child. I was supposed to have exercises twice a day. She did them three, four times a day. She'd heat oil on the stove in a little dish. Then she'd rub my leg with oil. I remember her coming to the school during lunchtime; she'd rub my leg with oil, make me do my exercises. She was doing that for my own good, but the other kids always made fun of me because my mother was always there.

Ted Kellogg contracted polio in Westfield, MA, in 1943 when he was five and a half years old.

I was transferred to a hospital-school facility, and my memory of it is hearing forties music blaring on a radio in the room where they put hot packs on me. The heat would loosen the muscles, and then the physical therapists would stretch your muscles to prevent or correct muscle contractures.

There was some brutality in the way that people were treated. There was a particular nurse who was verbally abusive. A lot of kids got head lice. We'd be taken into the bathroom, and some foul-smelling stuff poured on our head, and then a fine-toothed comb would be rammed through our hair to get rid of it. It was never done kindly, like your parents would.

I stayed in bed constantly. They didn't get me up for quite a while, and I broke several bones falling out of bed, playing, as kids are wont to do.

There was a separate school building. They would push the children out onto the lawn for recess, and it was on a steep embankment. This was in the days of the old rickety wooden wheelchairs with the springs under the seats and no brakes. I started rolling down the steep embankment, so I leaned over and tried to stop one of the wheels with both hands. The back of my head hit a tree, knocked me out cold. I went down the bottom of the hill, over a stone wall and out into the middle of the road where a bus had to come to a screeching halt in order to avoid hitting me. I was unconscious for over twenty-four hours.

Beatrice Yvonne Nau contracted polio in Bremen, KY, in 1943 when she was fourteen years old.

I was in Louisville at a crippled children's hospital. Sister Kenny had just visited, and they had to remove all of the iron lungs because Sister Kenny didn't approve of them. They did hot packs on my chest and my bladder. I had a male physical therapist. He put me in a warm water Hubbard tank. I was quite embarrassed because I had a very small t-strap on to cover me, and a small thing around my breasts. It was transparent when wet, so I was mortified. He was a very professional gentleman, and there was always someone around. It was not a one-on-one situation ever.

I went to the Sigma Gamma Hospital, which was the hospital school. I went in December of '43 and got out in June of '46. The minute I arrived, the nurse pulled me down to the footboard and said, "We keep our feet on footboards here." When dinner arrived, she fed me rutabaga. I said, "I don't eat that." She said, "We eat everything here." She was a very sadistic woman. She fed me all my meals until I was able to feed myself, which I tried to do as soon as possible. The physical therapist that I was assigned to was a young woman who had polio. She had scoliosis, but she walked and could use her arms. She was wonderful. She would stretch my muscles like nobody's business. I'd get tears in my eyes, but I still looked forward to my time with her because she was just a nice person. She remained my friend until she died a few years ago.

Edna Hindson contracted polio in Lake City, FL, in 1946 when she was six and a half years old.

At Warm Springs the first few nights were a nightmare because they didn't have room in the children's ward. They placed me in a teenager ward, and they delighted in tormenting me, making fun of me when I cried because I was separated from my mother.

We did not have any toys at Warm Springs. You played with what your parents brought. There was no equipment on the grounds to climb and swing. They had the walking bars once you got a brace. My father would not allow me to be just kept in a bed like so many of the other children. He got doctor's orders where I could get in a wheelchair and travel all over that huge campus.

The staff were too busy to pay much attention to me. Some family members brought me some oranges. After they left I was so frustrated, I took those oranges and smashed against walls. The walls were painted white, but nobody seemed to notice my destructive behavior.

I had very little treatment. They were not doing that much; I was just being housed there. It was always, "Well, when you get your brace." I had to wait and wait for that brace. I would go by the brace shop just about every day, and I'm sure they got tired of me coming there asking if my brace was ready because I wanted to go home. They did not know what to do with all of us. They were so backed up, and back then people in institutions or hospitals didn't have daily treatment.

THE 1950s

Ken Handal contracted polio in Brooklyn, NY, in 1951 when he was eighteen months old.

In 1951 I contracted a high fever. My parents took me to Kings County Hospital, where I was diagnosed with polio and I was quarantined with other polio patients. I became paralyzed in my legs and arms. I never had an iron lung.

My parents weren't allowed to see me. They would go up the fire escape and look in the window at me. They thought I was not being well treated, but they couldn't get me out. My parents had a cousin who knew a nurse at the hospital I was in. They paid this nurse $500 to smuggle me out of the hospital. They put me in a car, under a blanket in the back seat, so that people wouldn't see me. They took me out to Sister Kenny in New Jersey.

Siddequeh Wills-Foster contracted polio in New York, NY, in 1952 when she was six months old.

When I was six months old, I wasn't using my right leg. I had a fever for about three days. A doctor who came to the house didn't know what was wrong with me and gave me penicillin. My parents took me to another doctor who told my mother, "Your child has polio."

People used to stare a lot when she would bring me outside. They would ask, "What's wrong with your baby?" The bus drivers would let us ride for free. I didn't really date anyone until high school. I was always made to feel that I wasn't datable because there was "something wrong" with me.

Richard Rosenwald, M.D., contracted polio in Framingham, MA, in 1956 when he was thirty-two years old.

My wife, my daughter and I all got polio in 1956 even though there was a vaccine available. There was a shortage of the vaccine. I didn't want to use the black market to get it. Our pediatrician was in Newton; we were living in Framingham. He was forbidden to use Newton vaccine for anybody who wasn't a Newton resident.

I went to a meeting on Friday evening and developed a very severe headache. By Sunday I was feeling sick and my wife, Marsha, was starting to feel ill. Sunday night I was having trouble walking and urinating. Monday morning we called the doctor, who diagnosed the possibility of polio, and made arrangements for us to go to the hospital. My brother-in-law took us. He had to help me in. Marsha walked, which is kind of ironic, because she never walked again after that. We had spinal taps and were admitted. We ended up in iron lungs, side by side. A few days later, our nineteen-month-old daughter was admitted with polio.

It was uncomfortable and occasionally I had the sensation like I was falling. It's a big metal tube with a stretcher-like bed and it rolls in and out with a round area that has an opening for your head, and it seals around your neck. It's noisy; you hear it pumping. It creates a negative pressure that causes you to breathe in and then cycles out. You can move your arms and legs a little bit. There's a mirror-like thing on the top so you can see a little bit around you. It's not a great place to be, but keeps you alive. There are portholes that nurses can put their arms in. They would put a bubble on the end and use positive pressure while they took us out to clean us up. We were transferred to a whole room full of iron lungs. Then I went onto a rocking bed. I can't remember how long it took for me to go from the iron lung to the rocking bed, but I was much faster than Marsha. Marsha was in for quite a while.

Edward O'Connor contracted polio in the Bronx, NY, in 1955 when he was ten years old.

The ambulance ride was great because you could look out the window. When I got to the hospital, there were mothers around and little kids wrapped up in blankets. No one told me anything about why I was there. It was a Catholic hospital. I'll never forget the Sister who ran the place. She ran that place like a boot camp, but they were so understaffed, that that was the only way they could possibly run it. Kids were coming in by the carloads.

We went in to an examining room. A couple of doctors came in. I was really starting to stiffen up. An orderly came in. I thought it was a doctor, but it was a male nurse. He says, "Okay, we're going to taps." We went upstairs into this room, and I was on a gurney. They said, "You can't move, because if you move, you can cripple yourself." They put a pillow under my head and one person held my head and another held my feet. There was no Novocain; they just went in. They did it a couple of times.

I was put in a large dormitory and the beds were stacked up like Boy Scout camp. On one wall, they had all the kids who had had surgery. Their legs were apart, and they put them in body casts up to the breast line. We used to call them the three-monthers. They did that for three months. They just stayed in bed.

The place was just full of kids. In my room there were about 50 or 60 kids and the ages ran from eight or nine to twelve years old.

At night, if you needed something, you had to yell out, and you wouldn't yell out, because then all the other kids would call you a baby. Not unless you were going to die, then you might call out.

They would throw pieces of wool into this machine. They'd have you on your stomach, and they would put hot wool on your back and down your arms, and then they would put plastic over that. That was the treatment.

After the fever broke, I remember them saying, "You've got to go to physical therapy." They wouldn't let you out of bed because the muscles are so weak, if you could walk, you'd start getting crooked. Your back would go or your legs. I could move, but I had a limp for a while. My back was the one that was really bothering me. I used to sneak out of bed and go to the bathroom sometimes in the middle of the night rather than call out. It would hurt, though.

I hope X-rays aren't bad for you. I had ten thousand X-rays. We used to call physical therapy the torture chamber. They had an inclined plane they would set and they would slowly move you up, a couple of degrees, and then you would sit there for a half hour. That would hurt. They slowly progressed it until they had you sitting up. When I would sit up, I had no strength because my back was weak.

Your parents or your brothers and sisters could come between one and three on Sunday. They just isolated you. You're ten years old, and you can't see your mother, you can't see your father.

A couple of kids died, but we were told, "Their mother came and picked them up during the night." Even at that age, I wasn't buying it. We used to talk about that. "Do you think your mother would come here in the middle of the night?"

Jody Leigh Griffin contracted polio in Anchorage, AK, in 1954 when she was three years old.

I caught polio when I was three years old in Alaska. My mother took me to the doctor. He said I had a virus. I didn't get any better. She took me back again. Again, he said I had a virus. After two weeks, she found I was running a very high fever and having trouble moving. She took me back to the hospital, demanded that the doctor who had examined me before not even be on the premises. They determined that I had polio.

I had respiratory failure and I was completely paralyzed. I was in an iron lung. They transported me from Anchorage to Seattle. They flew a jet from an air force base in Texas to Anchorage to transport me in the iron lung.

I ended up at a respiratory center that was a Catholic-run organization in Seattle. I was there six weeks to a couple months. I remember having a tracheotomy. I remember going into the operating room and it being green and shiny stainless steel. I remember them putting a cloth over my eyes so I couldn't see. I remember being in the iron lung, still having the tracheotomy, and I wasn't supposed to talk. I couldn't unless I covered the hole, and they were always scolding me because I wanted to talk.

From the iron lung, I went to a rocking bed. It's like a seesaw, and it would raise me, lower me. It encouraged my lungs to inflate, deflate.

My parents started taking me to Warm Springs, Georgia. I was five, and I was in the hospital there six months. My parents moved to Warm Springs. Dad worked down there. I was alone for a while, from the time they took me and left me and then to come home and to move. They allowed me to go home Christmas Day for a few hours.

I have a lot of good memories of Warm Springs because I went there every year during my childhood. There was only one person-related bad memory. The head nurse of the children's ward was woman who did not like children.

My mother was a thorn in her side because my mother always advocated and paid attention. My mother did my laundry, and this nurse would tell the aides to use my clothes to dress whoever else. Half the kids in the ward were wearing my clothes. That didn't go over good. One lunch they served asparagus. When this nurse came to bring the vitamins, I had eaten everything on my tray except the asparagus. She told me I had to eat that asparagus, or she would take something away. I cried after she left. There was a maid bustling around. She was like, "What's the matter, honey child?" I told her.

She said, "Oh, don't you never mind. I'll eat it for you. She'll never know." She took the dish and put it in a drawer of the dresser. The nurse came back and said, "Did you eat it?" I said, "Yes." She asked me where the dish was; I burst out crying and told her. That maid got into trouble, and I had to eat the asparagus.

Stephen Burwick contracted polio in Worcester, MA, in 1954 when he was twelve years old.

I was in the hospital in Worcester at Belmont Home. I decided I had enough of this and I was going to leave. I shot up over the edge of the bed and crumbled on the floor and had to wait until somebody walked by to realize I wasn't on the bed anymore. Another time, my leg fell over the edge of the bed and I had to wait to have somebody pick it up. I'm not even sure I had the strength to sit up myself. I improved very gradually. Around Christmas time, the doctor said I would be going home in about a month. They were going to teach me how to walk again. I would be going home with a brace on my back and on my leg and crutches and have to do exercises and physical therapy at home. I had to learn how to pull myself up and walk between parallel bars and then with crutches and then upstairs and trying to get on a school bus and get off a school bus. It was just exhausting.

Margaret Alford's daughter, Peggy, contracted polio in San Diego, CA, in 1953 when she was eighteen months old.

I was living in San Francisco in 1953. My eighteen-month-old child, Peggy, contracted polio in the summer. We were living close to a naval officer who contracted polio about three days before Peggy got sick, and he died. In the meantime, we were ready to leave San Francisco. My husband was a naval officer, and we were on our way back to San Diego. Peggy was running a very high fever. We didn't connect it to anything. I tried to stand Peggy up. She just collapsed.

We went to a pediatrician, and he said she had infantile paralysis. She was quarantined immediately in the San Diego hospital. We were not allowed to see her except through a glass partition.

As soon as she finished that quarantine period, we had to have a hospital picked out for her recuperative treatment. We started in the Seventh Day Adventist Hospital. Since they could not treat her on Saturdays and it was recommended that she have treatment seven days a week, we decided against that. We went to a children's hospital in San Diego, which we were very impressed with. She stayed there for six months.

There was going to be a tremendous charge for her care. My husband was a lieutenant in the navy, our income was extremely small, and we had three children. We contacted the March of Dimes, and they said they would take care of everything. It was phenomenal. We never got a bill.

Peggy's hospitalization was probably one of the hardest things of my life because her father and I could see her for one hour, one day a week. The emotions were incredible on our end. She had no idea what was happening to her. The nurses and the aides fell in love with her and were marvelous to her.

She had the treatment of the hot packs on all of her limbs. She couldn't move anything. She could move her head and speak.

We saw improvement. Her legs began to come back. Her right arm seemed to be the most affected. At the end of six months, we took all of her best little clothes out there, dressed her up beautifully, and she walked out of the hospital on her own.

I had to take her back to the hospital three times a week for therapy. There was water exercise. There was traction exercise. It was tough on her because it was a real workout. March of Dimes paid for it all. It was just amazing. She wore a sling on her right arm always.

Norma Meehan contracted polio in New Bedford, MA, in 1955 when she was four years old.

I contracted from my cousin, and my brother also got polio. He was diagnosed with non-paralytic polio. My cousin died. She lingered in the hospital five or six weeks. I was playing with wooden logs, my brother was sitting on the floor with me, playing with his trucks, and I just lost all control of my body and fell backwards. My mother came running.

I was very weak. My mother put me to bed, and my father came home. The record shows August 5th when I was brought to the hospital, in 1955. My parents had to be checked out, too, and my brother was brought in. He was hospitalized a couple of weeks, and I was hospitalized twenty-two months. I was in the iron lung for three weeks.

My father tried his best, after I became sick, to find a doctor to vaccinate me. The third doctor said, "It would be like throwing it down the sewer. She's already got the symptoms."

The hospital became like my home. My parents were not well off financially, and they visited as often as they could, which wasn't that much. There were men who would come in and take things from children. My mother would get me comic books, and a man, he'd come in and go through my bureau and take toys and comic books. I had the fusion on my right shoulder. The parents of a teenage girl that was to the right of me were visiting with her, and the mother's on the opposite side of her bed, and the father's between her bed and mine. He just kept leaning back. He had his hands behind his back, and he was nudging my bed, and it waked me up, and an intense wave of pain, and I could barely speak. At that time they didn't have the buttons. You had to call, "Nurse." I didn't have enough energy to do that. The reason I got the impression he was doing it on purpose is he'd have this wicked smile.

Margaret Marshall contracted polio in Shrewsbury, MA, in 1955 when she was five years old.

I can remember looking at the March of Dimes posters and kids with crutches and braces and getting a feeling of terror. I would say prayers, "Oh, please, God, don't give me polio." I always thought about that because I came down with polio.

Some of the most disturbing memories of my polio experience revolved around the hospitalization, where today, the nurses could be termed abusive. I had to have a shot of something on a daily basis. I hated having it; it hurt, and I would temper tantrum. There was a nurse who said to me, "I'm going to roll you over. I'm going to change the sheet." They would roll you over, change one half, roll you to the other side, and change the other half. I cooperated with that because I thought it was a sheet-changing procedure. As soon as she rolled me over, what does she do but stick me with the needle. That made me so mad.

I remember another time kicking and screaming, and then being thrown into a hot tub of water. That was part of the regimen for polio people. The nurse carried me in the bathroom and then put me in this tub of water that was painfully hot.

When I finally got stuck in the hot water, I remember just sitting there just like a defeated person. I don't recall being abused, unless being thrown into a tub of hot water and being stuck with a needle when you don't expect it is abuse.

My father is a urologist and was on the staff at St. Vincent's Hospital, where I was hospitalized. My father came to visit me every day. I remember my mother coming just once. The doctor told my mother not to come. They said it was more upsetting when the mother would come to visit and then leave. The kid would cry and have a tantrum. It wasn't that it was hard for the mother or the child. It was hard for the hospital people to contend with these crying children. I remember being angry about it. I used to lie around wondering about my mother. All I could do was picture her at home with this little apron on in the kitchen.

Robert D. Blute, Sr., M.D.—father of Margaret Marshall.
When my daughter, Peg, contracted polio I was worried about all of my children. We had six or seven children then, and they'd all been exposed. The only one I was pretty confident of was my oldest boy, who got the vaccine. I went with my wife on April 12th, 1955 to Horticultural Hall. Dr. Salk was going to give his report on the effects and the benefits of the vaccine. Doctors were very excited because he thought the vaccine would bring about an 80 percent reduction in polio and he was right. He made the announcement that he had enough vaccine for only one—and they decided on the fourth grade.

Peg couldn't get it, just my older son. Two months after Salk announces the positive vaccine results, Boston has one of their biggest epidemics.

It was tough as a father, and as a physician. How come I didn't protect her better? I should have got the vaccine. I probably could have gone to one of the pediatricians.

My sister-in-law came down with polio, and Peggy was with her. When I came home from the office one afternoon, Peggy had all the signs. Our pediatrician put her right in the hospital, and all the other kids went to the ER. They'd give them passive immunity by giving them gamma globulin.

Peg was the first case in Shrewsbury, and in Worcester County, and it was followed by ninety other people.

A week after she was in the hospital, I remember driving down our street and saw an ambulance about four houses up. I said, "Gee, I hope that's not the little kid that plays with her." It was the kid's father with polio. It was a tough summer. We didn't see any neighbors. They wouldn't walk in front of our door. They would go across the street. Children seemed to disappear. There were a lot of kids in that neighborhood, and when she was in the hospital, they were not around our house. We were a pest house, a plague house. No one visited. We had to keep our children more or less confined, too, because we didn't know.

Gloria Smothers contracted polio in Boston, MA, in 1955 when she was four years old.

I woke up and I couldn't move my arm. My mother took me to Boston City Hospital. They told her I was constipated and to give me an enema. The next day I couldn't move my whole left side, so she brought me back. As she was bringing me back, I started not being able to move anything. They again told her I was constipated and I needed an enema. She told them, "There's something wrong with my daughter and I'm not moving."

The doctor examined me and told my mom I had infantile paralysis. They took me up to a big room with a lot of people, and they stuck me in this machine that looked like a round barrel; my head was out and the rest of me was in it. I couldn't feel anything except my mouth running and my head used to move back and forth. I was in the iron lung for four years.

Very nice nurses would sit by my little bunk. We were all in this one big room, the iron lungs on one side, and the other little kids that didn't need iron lungs were on the other side, moving and playing.

I found my hospital experience very positive because the nurses talked to me every day; they read books to me.

Lawrence "Larry" Lubin contracted polio in either Massachusetts or New York in 1952 when he was twenty-two years old.

My wife and I were on a trip, and the theory is that I caught it in the waters in Cape Cod, but I got sick after we got home; she was sick first. I might have caught it from her, although she has no residuals that say that she has polio.

I had full-blown bulbar spinal polio, and couldn't move anything. I was in the respirator for three weeks. Then I went to a rehabilitation center for a little over a year. I do remember them not seeing much hope for me. I had an uncle who thought maybe gamma globulin would help, and he was able to get it from connections. It was hard to get, and I had massive doses. I don't know if that ever made any difference.

I remember quite clearly at six months being still totally paralyzed. I remember the doctors telling my wife, "Be prepared for somebody who is going to be pretty useless his whole life." Most of my recovery came between six months and a year.

Regina Brown contracted polio in Utica, NY, in 1950 when she was twenty years old and a senior in a nurses' training program in a hospital.

I was admitted to the hospital and I spiked a high fever. After spinal tap, it was diagnosed that I had polio. There were many cases of polio in our area, so I was transferred to where all these people were. I had to be put in an iron lung. It's like living in a tin can. They were much bigger than they are now. I was in the iron lung for eight weeks. It was scary initially. You have to breathe with the lung, and once you're in rhythm with that, you're all right. The only way anyone has access to you are these little windows on the side that reach into the machine. Only your head sticks out. Everything has to be done for you.

People were afraid to come in to visit because they were afraid we were terribly contagious. The people that did come were such dedicated people. The doctors didn't go home. They slept there. The nurses were fantastic. As winter approached, they'd even come in on snowmobiles.

You're gradually weaned from the iron lung. You come out for an hour or two and then you go back. You get so dependent on something breathing for you, that you think, "I can't do this on my own." You'd go back in the lung again when you'd start to have labored breathing.

When the acute stage is over with, they start treatment of hot packs, and then hot tubs and hot packs. Your muscles are very susceptible. If someone didn't know how to handle you, it would be very painful. The physiotherapy would be twice a day, and it would start out very gradual. I was affected from head to toe, so that everything had to be worked upon. I weighed 88 pounds, and it would be like lifting a board. It would take two people to maneuver you because you're so stiff.

The physio would go gradually. You'd go in a wheelchair and then you'd go on crutches. I didn't need any braces of any kind. You'd have a corset-type thing, with braces that would go up your back, steel rods that would keep you straight, and you'd work with that for a few months. Then that would be discarded and you would do as much as you could on your own. The hot packs and the hot tubs would continue.

Edwina Jackson contracted polio in South Carolina in 1954 when she was four years old.

My stepfather took me down south to see his family. I drank the water down in that area, and I had a fever by the time I got back home. I was put in the quarantine hospital in Belleville, New Jersey. I remember being put in a room by myself, with a washing machine in the room. Every day the doctors and technicians would come in, fill that washing machine with hot water, put in blankets that had been cut up, wrap my whole body in those blankets, and put me in an iron lung. I would be in that all day.

On the days that my parents would come to see me, they'd line myself and other kids that were there up in the solarium behind this glass, and our parents would look at us and talk to us like we were on display.

I'm really not sure who paid for my treatment. My braces came from the Kessler Institute, and the United Way paid for a couple of things for me. My care must have been underwritten by the Welfare Department because my mother had public assistance at that time.

My mother stayed with me every day while I was sick, and that took a tremendous toll. She was a very young woman when she had me—still a teenager. This really was something new for her.

Ernest Greenberg, M.D., was in training during the polio epidemics in the early 1950s.

I was an anesthesiology resident at Grasslands Hospital, which is the county hospital for Westchester County, the polio center for Westchester County, as well as Putnam County. I was at the hospital in 1952, and from 1953 through 1956. We were primarily concerned with airway management of polio patients with respiratory difficulties. Since we were anesthesiologists and did many spinal anesthetics, we also did lumbar punctures on patients suspected of having polio. Patients would come in with fever, sore throats, stiff neck, stiff back. We met with Neurological Service and with Ear, Nose, and Throat to decide whether a patient required tracheostomy— patients primarily with bulbar polio, in which the respiratory center of the brain was affected. We had many iron lungs, and had nurses suctioning these patients around the clock. Patients in iron lungs would have pooling of secretions because they could not swallow. These secretions would cause laryngeal spasm. They would become cyanotic, very blue, and then it was an emergency intubation. Before going into the ventilator or respirator, they should be brought to the operating room. A tracheostomy should be done over the endotracheal tube. The trach would be a little higher than usual because the trach tube had to be outside of the respirator.

There was a lot of depression amongst the young mothers, especially anxious for their small children. I found my role more one of a pastor than of a physician, especially the patients who were in iron lungs. They were very concerned about their children, as well as themselves, wondering if they'd ever get home again.

A small child, about five years old—who I was watching, stopped crying, turned cyanotic. Intubated him, transported to the operating room for tracheostomy and later died. It was a very stressful day, and the memory of that and the child's name remains with me forever. It really bothered me terribly for many weeks to see a small child that I was involved with that I could do nothing about, as far as saving him.

The 1960s and After

Justine Guckin contracted polio in Newington, CT, in 1969 when she was two years old.

My right leg continued to atrophy. It ended up being three and a half inches shorter than my left leg. When I was ten years old, I had an operation at Newington Children's Hospital. I was the first one in New England to get this certain operation where they lengthened the leg by putting a bar in the femur. They put two pins right above my knee, and two pins right below my hip, on the outside of my leg, and cut my femur bone in half, and then turned the bar an eighteenth of an inch a day. I was in the hospital from October until February. It was terrible. The bar was sticking right out of my leg. When they put the bar in, my knee got infected where the pins were. It damaged some of the muscles in the knee in order for it to bend, so the big therapy of the day was to bend the knee, and it hurt like—it was unbelievable. They took a piece of my hipbone out to replace the space between my femur, and pinned that together, then took the bar out and let it grow together. They took the pins out once the bones molded back together. But they never did anything with the muscle. They just changed the bone. I went back about a year later, and they stopped the growth in my good leg. My right leg is still a tiny bit shorter so that I could swing it underneath me to walk. I don't have to wear the big heel on the shoe anymore, which I did as a kid.

3

POLIO'S IMPACT ON THE FAMILY

Feelings of fear and guilt often gripped families in which polio was diagnosed. Because of widespread news accounts of polio epidemics and, after 1938, the fund-raising campaigns of the National Foundation for Infantile Paralysis (NFIP), many Americans were aware of polio's capacity to kill its victims or to leave them permanently paralyzed and crippled.[1] Children could see fear and anxiety in their parents' eyes following a diagnosis of polio. In his classic study of how fourteen Baltimore families responded to a case of polio, Fred Davis discovered that parents experienced powerful emotions upon learning that their child had the disease. Parents particularly worried about the capacity of polio to cripple its victims permanently. Many called to mind the images of poster children in braces or wheelchairs, or recalled friends or acquaintances who were disabled by polio. Parental guilt feelings were usually lessened by assurances from doctors that there was nothing they could have done to prevent the disease, by prayer and comfort from religious advisors, and by the sympathy of neighbors and friends.[2] In some families, however, guilt feelings were not so easily assuaged and they had a corrosive effect on the family.[3] Davis also found that many families came to feel that polio had separated them from the mainstream of American life. Many parents had themselves "felt pity, or even repugnance, toward crippled persons," and the possibility of their child living with permanent paralysis seemed "unjust and unfair," perhaps even "un-American."[4]

Early in the twentieth century public health officials often quarantined families in which polio occurred. Sometimes, however, fathers were allowed to leave to go to work. During the great 1916 epidemic in New York and the northeastern United States public health officials also tried to limit travel from infected areas to those not yet experiencing the disease.[5] By the late 1930s and 1940s physicians recognized that a significant number of those infected in any epidemic had a very mild or unapparent case of the disease. Thus, it was useless to quarantine the apparent or paralytic cases, which typically made up less than 10 percent of all cases.[6] If official public health quarantines declined

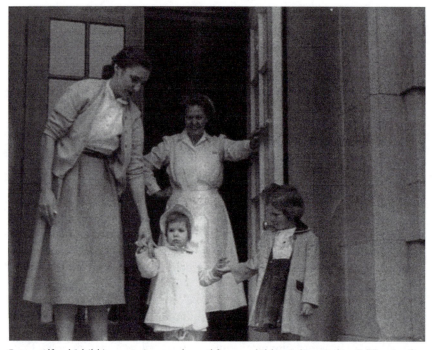

Peggy Alford (child in center) was released from a children's hospital in California after contracting polio when she was eighteen months old. Photo courtesy of Peggy Alford.

by mid-century, families in which polio struck often felt ostracized by their neighbors during the acute phase of the disease. Even if parents understood why others kept their distance, it hurt to be singled out this way.[7]

The long hospitalizations characteristic of both the acute and convalescent stages of polio created several problems for families. Parents and spouses of polio patients generally wanted to be at the bedside during the painful days of acute polio. Most, however, were kept away by strict no-visiting policies. It was hard, especially for children, to be so sick in a strange place inhabited only by gowned and masked doctors and nurses without comfort from their families. But it was also hard on parents forced to sit long anxious hours in waiting rooms or to stand outside hoping for a glimpse through a window. A few hospitals allowed occasional visits from immediate family, and some assertive families were able to visit the bedside, but most polio patients endured the pain of acute polio isolated from parents and family. The only exception to this separation in most hospitals came when doctors feared a patient was in imminent danger of dying; then a last visit might be allowed.[8]

Doctors often provided little information on a patient's condition or prognosis for permanent crippling. No doctor could give an accurate prognosis during the acute stage of the illness; there was simply no way to know how much damage the virus would do and how much of it would be permanent. However, Fred Davis also suggests that doctors were reluctant to make any predictions about recovery so as to forestall any recriminations later if the recovery should fall short. In addition, some physicians seemed to regard answering repeated parental questions as taking them away from their "primary tasks—diagnosis, prescription, and treatment." Although parents often tried to gain additional information from nurses and physical therapists, many remained frustrated by their inability to have their questions answered.[9]

Polio also imposed a financial burden on many families, especially before the March of Dimes developed its program to pay for patient care. Contemporary sources suggest that it cost between two and three thousand dollars to provide the first year's care for a serious case of polio. Costs continued to accumulate during the lengthy rehabilitation. The total cost sometimes reached $10,000 or more, and in the early 1950s it cost approximately $15,000 annually to care for a patient in an iron lung.[10] During the years of the epidemics, few families had health and hospital insurance. In 1940 only 9.3 percent of the population had hospital insurance and only 4 percent had surgical insurance. By 1950, just over 50 percent of the population had hospital insurance, but only 35.8 percent had surgical insurance. The low wages during this period meant that many families found it difficult to pay for care. In 1940 average annual earnings were just $1,299. By 1950 average annual wages had reached $2,992, but paying for a severe case of polio remained difficult for many families.[11] The March of Dimes paid for the care of many polio patients. Local chapters often paid for all or part of the care of individual patients, and the March of Dimes also paid for the care of iron lung patients and for the wages of doctors, nurses, and therapists during major epidemics. Families had to apply for aid, and local chapters were expected to provide assistance "to any family which would have to lower its standard of living by paying the total costs of medical and hospital care." The overall sums involved were substantial. In 1953, for example, the March of Dimes spent $29.7 million on patient care. However, that expenditure went to care for approximately 77,000 patients at an average of $385 per person.[12] Not all families who applied for aid received it, but even with March of Dimes assistance, the financial burden of caring for a polio patient through recovery could be significant.

The other financial burden of polio arose when an adult contracted polio, particularly if he or she was the family's major source of income. It was most often the loss of the father's income that affected the family financially. In some cases, the loss of income was only temporary because the wage earner was able to return to work quickly. In other cases, permanent disability precluded a return to work, or perhaps forced the individual to seek other less lucrative employment. A nonworking spouse sometimes found that she had to become the family's major source of income if her husband was unable to work. While a significant percentage of adult polio survivors returned to work following their recovery, even a temporary loss of income, coupled with the costs of polio rehabilitation, imposed financial losses on affected families.

In-hospital rehabilitation eventually came to an end, and virtually all polio patients returned home. But most were not fully recovered. The extent of paralysis could impose a significant burden on parents or spouses.[13] Some patients went home still dependent on an iron lung or rocking bed. Space had to be found, often in the living room or dining room, to accommodate all the medical equipment needed. Parents and spouses had to learn to care for a recovering polio patient and to administer necessary exercises. They also had to find ways to reintegrate their child or spouse into the life of the family. It was not always easy.

When the returning polio patient was a child, siblings sometimes found it difficult to adjust to the changed circumstances. The active, happy brother or sister often returned from the hospital unable to play as before. Sometimes the experience had changed them in other ways. They were more serious, more mature, and had left part of their childhood behind them. In addition, siblings sometimes resented the additional attention parents devoted to caring for their recovering child. In many families parents and siblings had to adjust to altered roles when a child with polio returned home.[14]

The return of a parent and spouse from polio rehabilitation posed its own set of problems. Adults were often more seriously paralyzed than children, and their return home meant major adjustments. Spouses usually became the primary caregivers, although older children often assisted. Mothers and fathers sometimes found it difficult to reassert parental authority following their long absence and with their new immobility. Severely paralyzed patients, especially those reliant on respirators, had to find ways to allow their spouses some independence if the marriage was to survive. Children had to adapt to having a parent whose paralysis prevented them from doing many ordinary things. In many cases, marriages withstood the strains and children adapted, but that was not invariably true.[15]

Families could assist returned polio patients to make a good recovery, but they could also, often unintentionally, put obstacles on the path to recovery and adjustment to a disability. Many families welcomed the patient home, encouraged them to continue their exercises, supported them if additional surgery was necessary, and helped them come to terms with any permanent paralysis. But other families, for whatever reason, found it difficult to continue the exercises, put unrealistic demands on the polio survivor to recover faster or more completely than possible, or failed to adjust to living with a person with a disability.[16]

Polio's impact on the families of patients varied tremendously. The severity of the paralysis, the length of hospitalization, the extent of the recovery, the adjustment of the survivor to his or her disability all affected how the polio survivor was reintegrated back into the life of the family. But the strength and cohesion of the family, the relationships between various members of the family, and the pre-polio family dynamics also impinged upon the polio survivor's reentry into family life and the response of the family to polio. Whether the impact was great or small, no family escaped unchanged when polio paid a visit.

THE EARLY YEARS

Ruth Esau contracted polio in Cass City, MI, in 1919 when she was two years old.

When I had my son, I was not a natural mother. I couldn't nurse him, I had no milk, and I couldn't satisfy him. One weekend, I took him back to the hospital and said, "You take him. I can't do anything with him." A younger doctor said, "I think you have a hyper baby. I want you to read Dr. Spock," and it helped me a little bit. Little by little, Eric grew to be a fine person. We had three children. Eric first, then Mary Beth, and then Ann Jean. Eric once told his godmother, "I don't know if you've noticed, but my mother has trouble walking." When I went back to teach, he was in the sixth grade, and he was a little ashamed. He was very quiet, but he never would say "Mom." He'd come into my room for art. He was sure that they didn't think I was his mother. If Eric were to hear that, he would dispute it. Mary Beth, the middle one, not at all. She'd just say, "Oh, Mom, Mom, Mom," and her classmates, too, they all loved me. My youngest was embarrassed. She was in kindergarten, and we combined for music class. She hoped nobody knew that the teacher playing the piano was her mother. She tried to cover up that I was lame. She'd walk in front of me. I'd say, "Ann, I can't step." She'd say, "Well, I'm just trying to fix it so no one sees you, Mom."

THE 1930s

Joan Rugh contracted polio in Bell Vernon, PA, in 1937 when she was eighteen months old.

I have two older sisters. As adults, I asked them how they felt about my having polio. One sister said she remembered sitting on the side of the table, and she would watch my mother do the exercises on me. She said, "I was probably sitting there waiting for her to get me something to eat." My other sister told me that they never felt that it was a burden to them, or never felt that they were being denied time. My oldest sister told me that for years she worried that she was the one who made me get polio because she dropped me on the sidewalk. She picked me up and I was okay, but within days I started to get sick. She always felt that if she hadn't dropped me that I might have not had polio. My mother finally convinced her not to think that way, that it was probably something that just couldn't have been helped.

Alice Cote contracted polio in Attleboro, MA, in 1935 when she was twenty-two months old.

My mom died while I was in the hospital and when I went home it was just my sister and my dad. My brothers were off at the war. I got bounced from one relative to another for many years, because I had to do ten exercises, ten times each, twice a day. There was never anybody who wanted to spend that much time helping me, so it got to be too much for this relative, my father would have to find me another place to live.

My dad got remarried. He told me once that he married because he felt that I needed a mother, someone to take care of me. She used to abuse me. I'd ask if I could go to the movies on Saturday, she'd say, "Well, if you polish the furniture, mop the floors, do the dishes, then I'll see." I'd do it, and then she'd tell me, I couldn't go. We always ended up on Saturday, noontime, with me on the floor, her 180 pounds sitting across my stomach, and her beating on my head with her fists, and then she'd walk out the door.

We lived in a duplex, and the woman that rented the other part of the house used to knock on the door and say, "Alice, are you all right?" I'd say, "Yes." She wanted so bad to turn her in to help me. She was a young widow with two small boys, and she was afraid of not having anyplace to live if she turned the landlady in for beating on me. That went on for about three years. I was deathly afraid of my stepmother. I didn't get over that until I was well into my thirties. If I saw her somewhere, I'd start shaking and crying.

The abuse finally stopped when my aunt asked me if I wanted to come to her house for Christmas. My stepmother said I couldn't go. My father said, "Why can't she?" She said, "Because she's got to do the dishes, and she's got to set the table, and she's got to—"

My father said, yes, I could go. When I was at my aunt's and uncle's I talked in my sleep. My uncle found out through what I was saying in my sleep that my stepmother had been beating me. I had never told a soul. I never even told the minister at church. Later the minister told me, "I always knew there was something wrong, but you never would say a word." The only one who ever knew anything was the woman next door, because she heard it.

My aunt and uncle decided that they would keep me. My father used to come Friday night right after work and pay board for me.

One day my younger brother came to where I was living and said, "I think you need to be with this other aunt and uncle." My uncle had tried to get fresh with me, and my aunt didn't want me there anymore. I went to this other aunt and uncle's in another town. This aunt and uncle were in their seventies, and they couldn't help me with my exercises. My brother came over there one night and said, "I think it's time you go back where you belong, with your sister and our father." He dragged me out of there and took me to my sister's house, and she wasn't very happy. My first year of high school, I'd been to four high schools. Nobody wanted the responsibility of helping. The biggest thing I missed out on in life is not having a mother.

I was always like a magnet to people to abuse me. I went through some counseling; I stuck with the same counselor for eighteen years. I asked him one time how come I always find myself falling into these relationships? He explained to me that it really began when I went into the hospital when I had polio. He said that I didn't have control of my body, and I was operated on, poked and probed. He said that's abuse of a sort. I got so used to the doctors and nurses doing whatever they wanted to me that I would say, "Okay. Do whatever you need to with me, and maybe I'll be better after."

George Durr contracted polio in Peekskill, NY, in 1931 when he was eighteen months old.

We were at Camp Smith in Peekskill, New York. I have a brother and a sister, and we all shared a banana that day. That night when we come home, I complained of pain in my neck. I was then brought to Grasslands Hospital, which is now Westchester County Medical Center. We were quarantined, because they didn't know how polio was transferred to other people. I was there for approximately four years. I recall many people being sick and many of them died.

My parents were only allowed to visit on Sundays, and they would bring toys, but the toys were sterilized and you couldn't get them for another day or so. My mother and father came in wearing white sheets. It was some kind of a gown that was actually frightening to the people who were there.

My father finally told the doctors that they weren't doing anything for me and that he planned on taking me home. I was around five years old at that time. I remember leaving the hospital, and I could not walk. I was completely paralyzed from the neck down. They had to strap me into the car. This was my first experience being outside—seeing trees and corn. The ride home was very exciting. It was just amazing to see houses and roads and cars. It was just an unbelievable sight to a five-year-old kid who had been literally strapped or locked into a bed his whole life.

When I got home I met my brother and sisters for the first time. They weren't allowed in the hospital. I didn't know who they were. The only people I knew were at the hospital.

THE 1940s

Ted Kellogg contracted polio in Westfield, MA, in 1943 when he was five years old.

I have one sister three years older than me and my brother is two years younger than me. I was close to my brother but not my sister. My having had polio might have been the major cause for alienation between my sister and me. We're estranged now. Her childhood was filled with Teddy this and Teddy that, because Teddy had polio.

I didn't spend much time at home with my family, though. I was in the hospital or living at the Canton hospital school most of my childhood. I was home for about a year and a half between being discharged from the hospital and enrolling in Canton. I was sent home with heavy leg braces from foot to waist that they thought I had to have on every day, and it was just a struggle. I had a back brace that I had to put on. Rehabilitation didn't exist, so I was not taught to do anything for myself. I just laid there like a lump and let people dress me. I tolerated braces when, today, I would have said, "Don't be ridiculous. If I'm not going to walk, I'm not going to wear braces."

When I came home from the school in Canton, my brother and I would basically team up against my sister and tease her and call her names. It was because she was older than we were, and both of my parents worked, so she was left "in charge" of us.

Ellen Balber contracted polio in Brooklyn, NY, in 1949 when she was six years old.

I was living in Brooklyn, New York, and my whole family was quarantined, not only my immediate family, but I lived in a four-family house that was attached to another four-family house, and all my aunts and uncles had apartments there, as well as my grandmother and grandfather. All my cousins were quarantined for a brief period of time. They were told to stay in and not make any contact with other children. My family was really ostracized for a little while.

My family was very disappointed by my recovery. They were happy that I was alive. I had bulbar polio. People don't even notice unless I'm wearing shorts, or a short skirt, which I very rarely do. My father was obsessed with physical beauty. If he saw I was limping he would walk in front of me and imitate my limp to make me stop limping. That was a very cruel thing to do. It probably did make my limp less because I was very well aware of it. It also made me self-conscious. In my teen years, I did not date much because of it.

My calf did not develop, so I had a very thin right leg and a normal left leg. My father decided that I should get a prosthesis that would fill out the calf of my leg. It was made with felt, covered with leather, and you wore it over an elastic stocking, and then you put a regular stocking over the elastic stocking. It was not a pretty sight. I wanted people to see me as I was. I thought it would be very uncomfortable to then take it off and show people something else. My father likened it to a woman who has her breast cut off and uses prosthesis for a breast, so that equated this with sexuality. I wore it for many years. I wore it the day I got married. It was a very unhealthy thing, and it made my handicap something that made me less. It robbed me of self-esteem, and my insecurity as a woman fed that. My father thought that no man would ever be attracted to me if I didn't have two normal legs.

I married a man who I was besotted with. I had just turned twenty. I don't know that we ever discussed my having had polio in depth. He knew I wasn't perfect, but it didn't seem to matter, which I find interesting to this day, because I'm so used to men like my father. My brother was like that, too. My brother—years later, when I was in my thirties—told me that he didn't think he could ever marry a woman who wasn't perfect or who had a deformity. That was after I was divorced from my first husband. I got divorced, and I thought that was really kind of terrible that I should have married the wrong person, but he wanted me. In those days, people did marry very young, but I was kind of afraid that my father might be right. I'd better grab while the grabbing was good. I did love him. I have been married to another man now for fifteen years.

If I didn't have polio I might have adopted my father's values. He died quite young—the rabbi was going on and on about his virtues, of which there were few, and my aunt said, "Why doesn't he just say he always looked good and he always smelled good." Because that's really all he cared about. I don't know that he was introspective in any way, and I suspect having polio made me that way.

Having polio and my family's response to it did color my perspective of who I was. It took a long time for me to overcome those feelings, and to this day a fervent wish of mine would be to have two good legs. When my children were born, the thought that they would never have polio and that they had two good legs was the most wonderful thing for me. I'm sixty years old, and I still wish I had two good legs, so obviously it's had a tremendous impact on my life.

Beatrice Yvonne Nau contracted polio in Bremen, KY, in 1943 when she was fourteen years old.

When I was nine years old, my sister was born. I fell in love with her. I was responsible for her a great deal. My mother and stepfather drank a lot, and they would go out in the evenings and leave me with her. She was four when I got polio. I wasn't able to see her, which really broke my heart because I felt as if I was deserting her.

My two daughters were a little embarrassed about my having had polio. The older daughter more than the younger. I was more comfortable with myself by the time Pam came along. With Kim, I was still staying in the car as much as possible and pretending I wasn't disabled. We'd go to drive-ins a lot. When I went out with my husband, Chet, he would pick me up and carry me up steps if he wanted to go someplace. He didn't seem the least bit embarrassed. He didn't avoid flirting in my presence, and how many of those women he eventually went to bed with, I don't know. He made me feel just worthless. I said I would marry Chet because I was thrilled about getting a proposal and because it was him. He was very sophisticated, and he'd been around plenty, but I just felt as if he would be the person to take care of me because he knew everything. Also, I didn't feel as if anyone would want to marry me, and I was flattered that he did.

Rick Spalsbury contracted polio in Oklahoma City, OK, in 1945 when he was two years old.

My parents were Christian Scientists. I never got any treatment. Christian Scientists believe that a supreme being can change anything and that prayer is the answer to everything. Medicine is not used. My parents didn't want to talk about my polio. It was ignored. Polio affected my legs. I walked on my hands and dragged the lower half of my body, up until I was six. Gradually I just started walking like everybody starts walking, a little bit—you fall down, and you get up, and it was just later in life, for me. Nothing in my life has ever been normal. My parents were embarrassed about me. They didn't want to have anything to do with any of it. Or me.

My parents said, quite a few times, that they wish I died. I'm not sure that wouldn't have been a better thing.

I'd come crawling through the living room, when they had company, and the subject would change, as to why I wasn't walking and what was wrong. They didn't want anybody to know about it. It's something that's contagious, and nobody wanted to be around it, for fear of catching it. They would put me in the closet when they had company.

Arlene Jordan contracted polio in Maine in 1947 when she was twenty-two years old.

I was working for Western Union Telegraph Company when the Island of Bar Harbor, Maine was on fire. They began to evacuate people to Ellsworth, Maine where I was working. There were many people standing at my counter wanting to send telegrams to let their relatives know that they were off the island. This went on for several days. I would work until 2:00 in the morning, and I would go home to get some sleep. I was so revved up that I couldn't sleep at all. So I'd go back to work at 3:00 A.M. I was tired and must have come into contact with someone in the crowd who had polio. Because so many people were displaced, we took a family in our house, which necessitated my sister and I sleep together. Our theory is that I had the virus first, and gave it to her. She was only five years old at the time. It was terrible. She was like a child of mine. She was quarantined, so I couldn't go in the room.

Samuel McKnight contracted polio in Connecticut in 1949 around the time of his birth.

My mother contracted polio the summer of 1949, and I was born with polio July 30th, 1949. There are other family members that had it, but I think the two of us had the most severe inflictions. My mother passed away from polio on September 25th of 1949, so she died approximately seven weeks after my birth. I was raised by my grandparents.

When my mother passed away, it was very difficult on my grandmother. My mother was eighteen years old. It was very difficult for my grandmother to overcome that. My father had a lot of difficulty, and eventually, moved out of the area. He was devastated from the loss of his wife and my affliction.

The 1950s

Priscilla Dewey Houghton contracted polio in Millis, MA, in August of 1955 when she was thirty-one years old.

I had three children. I know the exact day and what we were doing. It was a big epidemic, and 1955 was the last one.

We were so afraid for the children all the time. My daughter had actually had the vaccine that spring of '55. But the boys, who were younger, had not, and a friend took them up to another house in Millis and kept them away. We were having a hard time handling the whole thing. My son, when he went through therapy, said how deprived he felt by having his mother taken away from him at that stage of life. He was five.

I was at home, but I couldn't do anything. They'd come in and want to play or talk. I could talk, but I was just totally exhausted all the time. You're so tired that you can't move. The exhaustion goes on for years. It took maybe five years to get back.

We just couldn't do as many family things together. After polio I started doing a lot more intellectual things. I started writing these plays that the children performed. There's a director who lived near us, and for children in our town, I wrote plays for them and musicals and lyrics. We had this very theatrical life. It was quite an extraordinary gift from polio to me to get me back into a different world that way, but it wasn't a physical world; it was an intellectual world. It was very rewarding; it's been my life since.

Emily Donahue contracted polio in Ithaca, NY, in 1953 when she was seven years old.

"I know I'm sick, I know I'm throwing up, but why can't my mother come? Why does she have to wear a mask?" That was one of the reasons why she took it off. She just said, "We're never going to be able to pull the wool over Emily's eyes with everybody all gowned all the time. She's going to know that there's something really bad going on instead of knowing that she's sick and she has to be in the hospital a little bit."

It was pretty obvious that I needed to be at home because I wasn't able to walk. The routine was not to go into the hospital for any kind of physical therapy; this friend of my mother's who was a nurse volunteered to work with me. She helped get me out of bed and try one step and then another step, and she was also very involved in bathing me and thinking of interesting things that I might like to eat.

I stayed in a bed in my parents' room. Both they and I, in different ways, were very overwhelmed with how unable they were to do anything for me. I started to be afraid of everything, and I actually still am. Most of the fear for me comes in the form of being afraid for everybody that I know, my children in particular. At that point there was a big change in my relationship with my parents, and a lot of it had to do with that they really couldn't protect me anymore. That innocence stopped, and I was really young for it to stop.

Steven Diamond, M.D., contracted polio in the Bronx, NY, in 1953 when he was thirteen years old.

My parents came almost every day to visit me in the hospital. When I went home, my mother helped give me physical therapy, and she was a working person, so she'd do it early in the morning. I think it destroyed the relationship with me and my brother. I was thirteen. My brother was ten. My parents did the best they could do for him, but there was a lot of resentment about me getting so much attention. I went on to be a rather good student, and he didn't. We have a terrible relationship. We took my mother to our home in Florida for the winter. We were hoping she would live there. She couldn't stand it. She said, "I'm going home. The people here are too old." My brother said to my wife, "You only want Mom in Florida so she can push Steven in a wheelchair." My having polio and his resentment about it has ruined his life. It's important to understand that the shock of that illness to a family in those days was like the ultimate in devastation.

Fred Bloom contracted polio in Boston, MA, in 1955 when he was thirty-eight
years old.

My son David, age six, was hospitalized in July, and he went to the Children's
Hospital. He was diagnosed with non-paralytic polio. Two weeks later, my
brother Herbert, age thirty-two, contracted polio. Twenty-four hours later, I
seemed to be getting symptoms. I talked to my doctor and told him that I had a
high fever and achy, and he said, "Grab the first cab and come down," to Mass
Memorial. I only had it from my hip down to my toes, my left leg. Herb, on
the other hand, was getting paralyzed in his legs and a little later moving up,
and then ten minutes later he said, "They're taking me to the Haines Hospital."
They rushed him over because he had to go into an iron lung.

Edith was a therapeutic dietician at the Mass Memorial, and I later married
her. After contracting polio, my brother was a quadriplegic. My wife, Edith,
said, "We have to take care of Herbie," and I was shocked. It may be one
thing for a brother to take care of a brother, but for a sister-in-law, that was
pretty heavy stuff. We talked it over and she insisted. We made a decision to
build a house that would be able to fit the wheelchair. We knew we wanted
some private living; we were just newlyweds. The house was built on one
level. There were two bedrooms on the first floor, which was same floor as the
dining room, living room, and kitchen. Down a flight of stairs was a full-height
basement. We had two bedrooms down there, where Edith and I and later
our daughter, Linda, lived.

Ruthanne Werner contracted polio in Bradford, PA, in 1952 when she was eight
years old, along with her mother and three siblings. Only her father was spared.

My younger sister, Betsy, who was two at the time, first contracted polio
shortly after a neighbor boy, Joey, who had gone to the hospital with a diagnosis
of polio. My mother's memory is that we caught it from Joey. His parents
remember that they got it from us. They have their version and we have ours.

A week or two later, my sister Debbie went to the hospital and the same
day I went. Two weeks after that, our mother was diagnosed with polio. My
brother had some of the symptoms, but it never reached a point where they
felt he needed to be hospitalized.

I remember therapy hurting a lot. We cried during therapy. One therapist
said, "If you don't stop crying, I'm going to put you in the pool and hold your
head underwater." I couldn't stop crying. She did hold my head under water,
though not for very long. After that I was pretty scared of that therapist. I have
to give the staff some allowance for stress. I didn't suffer any physical damage,
but it was a scary place to be.

When we moved to Colorado, I went to Children's Memorial Hospital in
Denver, and it was like night and day. I have really nice memories from
Children's. The therapy was easier to deal with. I had a lot of visitors. That's
one of the advantages of being a preacher's daughter in a town where there is
a church in your denomination. My mom was in St. Luke's Hospital just across
the street; we could talk on the phone.

The hardest part was being separated from my family. I just wanted to go home. I felt lonely, although, there were some very kind people who helped. My father was just overwhelmed; three of his four kids and his wife all had polio. My mom has one bitter memory. She was feeling sick, and the doctor had come on Saturday, and it had been decided that Sunday morning she would need to go into the hospital. My dad went ahead with the church service. We lived in an apartment; it was part of the church. When she was being wheeled out, he could see it through the church windows. My mom thought that he should have canceled the service and gone with her. He thought his first responsibility was his congregation. They stayed married and a lot of things got worked out. When she tells it, she says, "He should have gone with me. It was the worst day of my life."

There's a picture that was taken of the family. Debbie, Tim, and Betsy were all there, just looking kind of scared. My grandmother had this weary look on her face, and my dad had a big smile—like he's got to be the on-top-of-things pastor. That's the saddest thing of all; my dad had to keep up a front like that.

Michael Masters contracted polio in Africa in 1952 when he was twenty months old.

My parents were missionaries, and we were living in Southern Rhodesia, Africa. An epidemic swept through the village, and four out of six of us contracted polio. My father and my sister got bulbar polio and died from it. My mother and I also got polio. I had some recovery in my arms, but my mother was paralyzed from the chest down. My two brothers did not get polio. Polio had a huge impact. Everything in my life was affected by it.

Once the condition was stabilized in Africa, they brought us to the United States because that's where the home church was, and it was an easier place to get medical treatment. I started out at Children's Hospital in Boston, but very shortly I was transferred down to Warm Springs Foundation in Georgia.

I don't remember much of anything up until ten, twelve. I spent a lot of time in body casts my first several sessions down there. When I came to the United States, my spine was a total S-shape, one of the curves being right next to my heart. I went into a body cast right away.

My mother was with child at the time we got polio, and she lost the child.

I was pretty active as a kid. I wasn't one to just lay around and mope, so I was up pushing myself around from the time I was little, and I had this tiny wheelchair, and I tore the rubber off my wheels going down hills. I had to spend a lot of time doing exercises. I have vague recollections of having to get on my crutches and walk on those, and having to do different exercises. I remember a lot of boredom. Where my bed was, I couldn't see out the window, so I tried to drill a hole through the wall so I could see outside.

Polio affected relationships with peers, with girlfriends, with growing up and being a man, with self-esteem, with physical ability to do things. It shaped virtually every part of my life. I use a wheelchair—I view life from the sitting position. I don't perceive things in the same way as other people do, simply because I've never looked at things from the perspective that other people have. I tend to be a little bit of a loner. I'm not unfriendly, but I'm not a garrulous person, either. I don't crave human company. I'm perfectly happy being alone. That's probably one of the biggest aspects of how it's affected me.

Neil Wells contracted polio in Epson, NH, in 1952 when he was five years old.

We were living in Epson, New Hampshire. I was admitted to the Margaret Pillsbury Hospital. My father had polio, and my sister. We were all admitted about the same time. My father died of it. My sister was left with minimal effect to her ankles. I was hospitalized from October until January. I remember from the initial polio when my mother came in and told me that my father had died. I've reconstructed a little bit of it from newspaper articles. My father was only alive for about three days, and was in an iron lung. My father's was the first death from polio at that hospital during 1952. The deathbed request he made was, "Don't send flowers to my funeral; give money to my family." That quote made the papers, and people started to donate. Shortly after my father passed away, the house that he had been building for my family burned. My mother and father bought the land and this barn. My dad had been a carpenter, so he converted it and turned it into a seven-room house. It was not quite done. There was no water system in it. A lot of people donated money, and some companies donated materials. There were a number of contractors that volunteered their time to install it and finish the house. After they had just started the work, it burned. All the volunteers' tools were lost. All of the donated building material was lost. It was put down as suspicious cause, maybe a short circuit. There was nothing in the house that could have been an ignition source. My mother always figured that somebody torched the house. They didn't want the polio spread any further. There was a tremendous response from people throughout the neighborhood and actually it ended up being the whole country. People donated things, from a week's worth of groceries to building materials, and they ended up putting up a whole brand-new house for us. Even the state prison, the inmates donated $155, and they were only making about 15 cents an hour, so that was quite a lot of money. The governor at the time donated the kitchen cabinets. For years afterwards, whenever my mother needed a babysitter, the neighbors were always there to help.

I used to go up to where the house burned down there and hang out. It was a nice piece of land. One day I was walking up to the old foundation. This was probably ten or twelve years later. A glint of light caught my eye. It was my father's war dog tags hanging off a tree. We had almost nothing that was his because everything was in the house and it burned.

Edward O'Connor contracted polio in the Bronx, NY, in 1955 when he was ten years old.

I was the youngest of seven kids and I think having polio made my family a little softer on me. They felt that I had been through a lot of stuff and they would give me more slack. Polio took a toll on my father, and my mother, too.

The year I got out of the hospital my father had a massive heart attack. He had high cholesterol. He lived for another eight or nine years after that.

Norma Meehan contracted polio in New Bedford, MA, in 1955 when she was four years old.

The day my family came for me felt like I was with strangers. I remember trying to turn my head to take one last look at the hospital, and I really couldn't do it because I had the back brace on. My family was shocked and in denial. I had to be strong and pretend I'm not crippled. I was six years old. My sister was probably three and a half. She kept coming over to the room and sticking her tongue out. My mother was getting frustrated because she was getting me ready for the day. I was laying there with no clothes on, on my stomach, and she had to get the back brace on. She went into a fit of rage because my sister wouldn't obey her. My sister was running around the apartment, and my mother was striking out, a leather belt. She was striking with the metal, holding the strap. My sister went under the bed, and my mother went around to try to stop her. She thought she was going to come out the other end. My sister stayed there. My mother went around to the other side, and my sister went into the closet. She got away. My mother turned her rage on me. I was struck over a hundred times. It left some scars. There were over a hundred on my rear end, buttocks. I bled. My mother put Vaseline on it. My father came by and asked why I was crying. My mother said, "Oh, it's just because—" At that point I felt betrayed, and I just closed in. In my late twenties, I told my mother, because she had a tendency to slap me, "You hit me again, and you'll never see me again." She never hit me again. It's just a matter of standing up to her.

THE 1960s

Justine Guckin contracted polio in Newington, CT, in 1969 when she was two years old.

My mom took it really hard when I got polio from the vaccine. Having polio was hard. When we'd go somewhere, they'd always have to think ahead, what are we going to do, will I be able to walk, or do they have to carry me? My mother used to bring me to healing sessions, like Billy Graham. One time we went to Rhode Island and we had to sit on the front stairs of the church in order to get in. We had to get in line early in the morning. My whole family went, but me and my mother were on the stairs. My father took the rest of my brothers and sisters to the amusement park for the day.

It was a financial burden at first. I was in the hospital having surgery when I was ten. My mother's phone bill was astronomical at the time, because I'd call home collect every day. I didn't know that until years later, because she never said anything to me about it.

My family has always been very supportive of me. They've all just treated me like everyone else is treated, and they helped me when I needed help.

Because I had polio it taught everybody in my family to learn to accept what you have and be happy with what you've got.

Margaret Alexander contracted polio in Missouri in 1970 when she was five years old.

I picked it up from another child that had the live virus. I had been vaccinated but was due for one more. I remember I was real tired, real sick. I went to the doctor. He gave me an antibiotic shot in my rear end, and by the time I got home, I wasn't able to walk inside the house. Mom carried me in, put me in bed and said, "Well, you're probably just a little weak," since I had been sick for about three or four days.

When they tried to get me out of bed, I couldn't walk. My parents took me to the University of Kansas Hospital. They had me in isolation because they didn't know what I had. They ran all kinds of tests, and then they figured out I had polio. The doctors were very surprised because at that time there was no cases reported. I was then transferred to Children's Mercy Hospital in Kansas City, and there I stayed for about a month. My mother stayed with me most of the time. My family could come in, except for when I was in isolation.

I remember that the nurses weren't nice at all. They were afraid to touch me. It was the same way at Children's Mercy. I had surgery done there, and the nurses were mean. When they come down to take the medicine, if you didn't get it taken, they would put it in your milk and make you drink it like that. They always just sat there and waited for me to drink it. I'd gag and spit. That was pain medicine, so from then on I didn't ask for pain medicine anymore.

I had physical therapy, and they did this electrical shock on my legs. Even though I was paralyzed from the waist down, it still hurt. I went home in a wheelchair. It was a good eight months later before I could get out of the wheelchair, and they said I never would.

My mom was pretty good. Dad didn't take it very well. He worked nights, and he wouldn't come to the hospital to see me. When I had surgeries, he didn't come at all. My mom didn't drive at the time, so Dad would always take us down there and drop us off until it was time to be picked up. He started to drink a lot. Polio changed a lot of things with my family. Everybody was affected with me being in the wheelchair. It changed my one brother because he acted up a lot in school. He got in trouble with the law. It also caused problems with money and the house. It was hard on my Mom trying to pay the hospital bills. Nobody helped.

4

LIVING WITH POLIO

Returning home to familiar comforts was only one of many steps polio survivors took to resume their lives following the end of their hospitalization. Living with polio meant finding ways to return to school or work. It also meant learning to live with a disability in an able-bodied world that expected the polio survivor to make whatever accommodations were necessary. It meant, as well, learning how to deal with unkind words, impolite stares, discrimination, and stigma. But polio survivors by and large persevered. They found ways to mount the steep staircases of mid-century schools. They convinced employers that they could work from their wheelchairs. They married, had children and raised families. In short, they found ways to live successfully with polio.[1]

For children with polio, returning to school was often the first challenge they faced as they began to rebuild their lives. Rehabilitation hospitals at mid-century usually tried to provide some kind of opportunity for youngsters to keep up with their schooling, but it was not the same. There were a limited number of subjects, and the pace of instruction was very different. Other children were tutored at home until they were ready to return to school. Most children whose polio kept them out of school desperately wanted to return to the class they had left. They wanted very much to avoid the stigma of being held back. Whatever the deficiencies of their interim education, the vast majority of polio survivors who were able to return to school resumed their education with their class.

Returning to school posed a number of challenges for young polio survivors. School administrators often raised the first hurdle. At a time when students with any kind of disability were rare in school, not all administrators welcomed back students with disabilities. Some pointed to physical barriers—steep staircases, the lack of elevators, inaccessible bathrooms—as reasons to exclude polio survivors. Others cited the discomfort teachers and other students would feel in the presence of someone with a disability. Polio survivors, however, found ways around the obstacles. Students who could negotiate stairs with

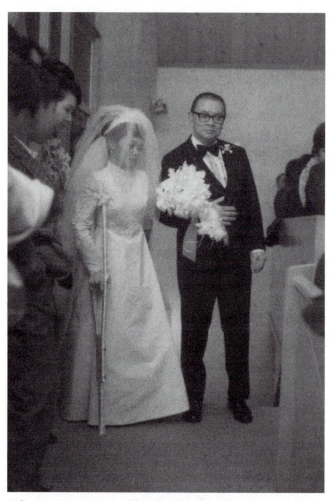

Polio survivor Noreen Abbott is shown on her wedding day in 1971. Photo courtesy of Noreen Abbott.

their crutches were sometimes allowed to leave classes early so as to move slowly to the next class. Fellow students carried their books. And in some schools friends lifted their wheelchairs from floor to floor. Because they recognized the importance of education for children with physical impairments, polio survivors and their parents made every effort to surmount the physical and social barriers thrown up by both private and public schools.

Polio did not impair cognition and polio survivors were often good students because they recognized that they would have to compensate for physical impairments by using their minds. Many became better students than they had been before getting sick. But if they were better in most classes, physical education classes posed another challenge. Some schools provided alternatives to students physically unable to take physical education, but polio survivors participated to the extent that they could.

Polio often put an end to athletic activity. For young men who had been successful athletes, the impairments of polio seemed particularly cruel. In a few cases, survivors recovered sufficiently to once again take up sports. Others became scorekeepers or athletic managers, which allowed them to maintain a connection with sports. And some focused on extracurricular activities where physical ability was less important.

School years were also the time when young men and women began to date. Dating in high school was fraught with anxiety under the best of circumstances. Entering the dating scene with an obvious disability was sometimes more than polio survivors could contemplate. Many of them, both male and female, went through high school without a date. Others, for whatever reason, were more successful in surmounting the cultural, social, and psychological barriers that kept so many sidelined.

College posed its own set of challenges. Most colleges in the fifties and sixties were as inaccessible as schools. However, many polio survivors realized that a college education would give them access to jobs that were less physically demanding. Polio survivors were often the first members of their families to go to college. In some cases they were helped financially by state departments of vocational rehabilitation. Polio survivors had to figure out how to live independently in a dormitory or apartment and how to negotiate the campus. As a result, the adjustment to college was often difficult. But they persisted. Some found relatively accessible campuses such as the University of Illinois. Others, such as Ed Roberts and his friends at the University of California at Berkeley, persuaded and even forced the university to make accommodations that allowed them to live independently and to earn their college degree. The efforts of these pioneers in finding ways to gain a college education eventually helped open doors to higher education for young men and women with many different disabilities. Although some polio survivors dated in high school and married their high school sweethearts, more dated in college. Both they and their potential dates were more mature, and their physical impairments seemed less of a barrier to intimacy.

Most polio survivors saw college as an opportunity to acquire skills they needed to compete successfully in the job market. Working, being able to support oneself or one's family, was vitally important to many polio survivors. Some adult polio survivors were able to return to their jobs after their recovery and rehabilitation. That possibility was dependent on several factors. First, the employer had to have kept the job open during the many months of recovery. Second, the polio survivor still had to be physically able to do the work. Third, the employer had to make necessary accommodations. Fortunate survivors had a disability that permitted a return to the work they had previously done and employers who welcomed them back. But many survivors discovered that their disability and the physical demands of the job meant finding different work. In seeking employment, they often encountered significant difficulty. In spite of national campaigns to hire the handicapped, many employers were unwilling to hire men and women with disabilities. Some were unwilling to hire the disabled because of prejudice. Others were unwilling to make the necessary accommodations. Still, because of their higher levels of education and drawing on the persistence learned during their long rehabilitation, most polio survivors who wanted to work eventually found employment. Only about 3 percent of polio survivors never worked.[2]

Like their friends during the post–World War II decades, polio survivors married and raised families.[3] Older survivors who were already parents when polio struck continued to raise their children even if from a wheelchair, a rocking bed, or an iron lung. Being a good parent meant much more than physical strength. For those not yet married when polio struck, the disease posed challenges in dating, developing intimacy, and making a commitment to marriage. Most, but not all, eventually found lovers and spouses.[4] Of course, not all marriages involving polio survivors were happy and successful. If the postwar decades saw a baby boom, they also saw increasing divorce rates. And just as polio survivors participated in the baby boom, so too, some of their marriages ended in divorce. Although the legacies of polio may have played a role in dissolving some marriages, the cultural and social factors that produced the high national divorce rates also affected the marriages of polio survivors.[5]

Going to school and college, working at a rewarding job, and finding a lover and spouse are often difficult even for individuals without significant physical disabilities. For polio survivors, the difficulty was sometimes magnified by the severity of their impairment, by the psychological consequences of polio, and by the expectations and prejudicial attitudes of teachers, employers, and lovers. The voices in this volume speak powerfully to the challenges polio survivors faced, the ones they surmounted, and the ones they did not.

1930s

Robert Lonardo contracted polio in Providence, RI, in 1935 when he was three years old.

We lived in a tenement house. We lived on the middle floor, and I used to get up and down the stairs like a dog. I'd be on my hands and knees. My father was a barber and had no talent for building anything. But why did they not have rails put in that house for me, just to go up the stairs?

I went to a "cripple school." It was a school for patients with entire paralysis because of some big epidemics. We all went to the same school from kindergarten all the way through the eighth grade in one classroom.

I always felt my mother never expected anything from me. I had to prove to her that I could be successful. Having polio broke my heart. I really wanted to be just like everybody else. As an adult, I had to be the best brace maker in the state, and I turned out to be. I am married and had five kids; inside of me always I felt I was never good enough. I think it was the reflection of what my mother felt about me.

David Rubin contracted polio in Brooklyn, NY, in 1935 when he was nine years old.

I was paralyzed for about six months. I remember sitting by the window, watching all the kids playing, and feeling badly that I couldn't join them.

Once I started to get my strength back, I became very active. In high school I had an afternoon job with a local grocery store chain where I drove a truck and delivered merchandise. One of my customers was on the third floor of a walkup, and I remember carrying cases of soda up to the third floor.

When America entered World War II, I enlisted with the Army Air Corps. I volunteered for gunnery. I thought that would be a quick way to get transferred overseas. Being Jewish, I was very sensitive to the issue of the Germans and the Holocaust.

I had to pass a number of tests, which were physically challenging like the obstacle course. I had to jump over a wooden wall. I had relatively short legs due to the polio. My upper body was quite strong. Coming around this bend I saw the wall and several of the officers who were running the program. I said, "Oh boy, I don't think I'm going to be able to get over that," but I tried. I ran as hard as I could and jumped, hit the wall, put my hands up at the top, but I couldn't get my legs over. I dropped to the ground, and the officer said, "You've got to get over this."

I said, "I don't think I'm going to be able to do that."

He said, "Go further back."

I went further back and I took another run, hit the fence, and tried to get my legs over. I couldn't get them over.

The officer said, "Go further back."

I said, "It won't make any difference because I'm not going to get my legs over."

He said, "You're going to do it because you have to do it."

I went way back. I hit the wall, put my two hands up on the top of it and it was like I was jet-assisted; I was flying over the fence.

Robert Huse contracted polio in Lowell, MA, in 1931 when he was six years old.

I was a hell raiser in prep school during my teens. I knew the full story about the polio. I was in the kind of denial that if I admitted how helpless I really was, I never would have gone out of the house. I was determined to have a life. That's why I went to prep school. I completely blew it by acting like an idiot, and got kicked out.

For one of my first auditions that I took in radio, I saw that there was no railing on the stairs. There were about fifty people there. You just line up, and you read something into a microphone, and then they separate the impossible from the ones that might make it.

When I saw the railing, I said, "That is not going to stop me." I waited until I saw somebody who looked really healthy, and I said, "You guys give me a lift?"

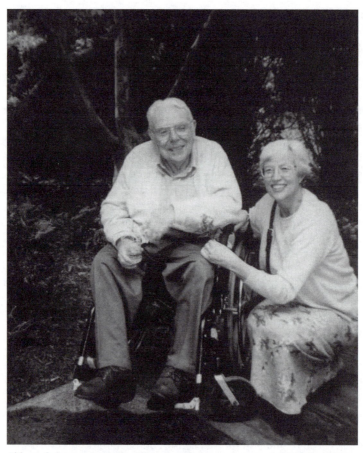

Although he contracted polio when he was six years old, Robert Huse persevered and grew up to become a popular evening radio disc jockey in New Jersey. He is pictured here with Margarete Arndt in 2000. Photo courtesy of Robert Huse.

I put my arms around their necks, hoisted myself up, and they dragged me up the stairs.

The program director said, "We're going to have these four audition for the management." They came out and said, "You stay." I had experience by then. I had worked at two other radio stations.

The program director had only seen me sitting down, so he didn't know that there was anything unusual about me at all. When I came into his office, he looked at me as if, "Is this the same guy?" He was very nervous, and this had thrown him for a loop. This was the first time that I ever ran into discrimination. Here he was offering me the job, and he began to say things like, "I don't know if this is the kind of a job you'd be able to do."

I said, "Are you offering me a job?"

He said, "Well, providing you can make it. Can you do the work?"

I said, "Well, I've worked at two other radio stations, and I've never had any complaints in that department. There's only one thing. You don't have a railing for your stairs. It's two flights up."

He said, "No, we don't."

I said, "Well, I'll pay to have a railing put up the stairs, because I really can't make those stairs."

He said, "We can't do that."

I said, "Why not?"

He said, "We have heavy equipment coming up the stairs, and it wouldn't fit because of the rail."

I said, "I'll pay any time you've got something coming up the stairs that's too big to go up that stairwell. I'll pay to have the railings taken off and put back on."

"No, we can't do that."

I said, "Are you telling me that for whatever it costs to put up a railing, that you won't let me work here now that you've seen that I'm on crutches?"

"It's not that at all, and I consider this discussion closed," he said.

I said, "Well, I don't. I want you to just tell me why you don't want to hire me."

He said, "I consider this discussion closed," and he got up and walked out.

Alice Cote contracted polio in Attleboro, MA, in 1935 when she was twenty-two months old.

When I went home during the war, my two brothers were overseas. My sister had a baby and was pregnant, and I had a half-brother, and my father, myself, and my sister's husband lived in this two-bedroom apartment. It was weird getting used to the ceiling being so close to me because the hospital ceilings were so high up. Having to go to school was a new experience for me. In the hospital all those years, we had a teacher who would stand up in front of us. She'd have a book on geography or spelling or history or arithmetic. It's the only four things we ever did anything with. None of us had books. She would talk to us. When I came out of the hospital, my father went to enroll me in September. The school board said I couldn't be put in the sixth grade. He said, "Well, she's already had five years." They didn't consider that what I had was formal education. They said that I needed to be put in first grade. My father fought with them and said he wanted to at least give me a chance. They came to an agreement. If I didn't pass it, then my father would start me back in first grade. He told me, "You were twelve years old. I wasn't going to put you in first grade because I didn't want you to be humiliated like that." I did pass that year, and I didn't feel the effects of trying to learn until I got to high school. I spent three years as a junior, just trying to pass the geography and history, but I did graduate.

George Durr contracted polio in Peekskill, NY, in 1931 when he was eighteen months old.

When I got home the first day, my father used his belt to strap me into the chair. He had a crib that he made where I slept. They wanted me to eat, and my father put me into bed if I didn't eat. He did it for my own good, but it upset my mother and it upset me. I finally did settle down and was able to eat and do what the family did.

About a year and a half later they wanted to know if I would like to go to school. I said, "I won't be able to walk to school." We lived about five blocks from the school. My brother would get a wagon, and I was brought to school with my brother and sister. The teachers would help me get into a chair, and I was gradually able to participate in schooling. I couldn't do many of the health and sports things, so I took that extra time to catch up with the rest of the students who were ahead of me in the first year. By the fourth year, my skills had developed to where I was equal to the rest of them.

My high school principal got me to be the scorekeeper and travel with the team. That was in eighth and ninth grade. That was a big boost for my morale to be with the sports heroes. Then I got to the local newspaper, and I would telephone in when we got home what happened.

In the tenth grade, I did my homework at those free periods I had. When I went home, I was always looking for something to do. My father had a shotgun that he didn't use anymore, so somebody put an ad in the paper that they would swap their band saw for a shotgun. With this band saw I started to cut out names for your house and paint it. I established a contract with Sears & Roebuck. I would make these signs for fifty cents and they sold them for a dollar. The kids would laugh, "How come you always got money in your pocket?" I said, "Well, I got a business. I work when I go home at night."

1940s

Bill Norkunas contracted polio in Worcester, MA, in 1944 when he was four years old.

I was in the iron lung for two years. When I was discharged from the hospital, I had to go back regularly. I can remember commenting one time, "How come I can't take this Easter recess and play with the kids?" The answer was because I had to go into the Children's Hospital. I went to summer camps for kids that had polio, where they had a structured environment and you got exercise. The only bad memory I have going to school is being in the men's bathroom and sitting in a toilet stall. Someone came in, looked to see who was there, and said, "Oh, that's Bill."

"How can you tell?"

"Well, I see the big shoe."

Another kid said, "Shhh. Don't say that."

That's the only comment that I ever heard.

I went to a Catholic school on the other side of town, and I would take public buses every day. The bus used to wait. If I was late, a passenger would get off and come up to my house because the bus would not go until I was on. My mother said, "I wonder how many people were late for work because they had to wait for the bus?" They never even thought of leaving without me.

My mother told me that the neighbor children were not allowed to play with me because I had polio. She said, "After we brought you back from the hospital, no one would play with you. The neighbors didn't allow it. You didn't have any friends. It was just you and your brother who was two years younger than you." She said, "But the garbage men would come to the house, and they would say, "Does Billy want a ride in the garbage truck? And they would take you out." She said, "That used to be the biggest source of excitement."

I didn't have any friends until I got a little bit older, when I could start playing sports, and then I excelled. I could throw footballs further. I could hit baseballs further. I could pitch better. The kids really accepted me because of my athletic ability. I've always worn a brace, though.

In high school I never saw having polio as a problem because I excelled. I received a gold award letter every year. I can remember a standing ovation from my high school. The kids were really supportive.

I always thought, if I didn't have polio, would I have more dates, or would I have been more popular with the girls? I remember one time having a date and bringing her out to a nightclub. I went to the bathroom, and when I came back, my date said to me "When you got up one of the guys over here came over and said, 'Who's the guy with the limp? I think I know his name.'" she said, "I started looking around for him. Then I realized he was talking about you. I just didn't see it."

I will tell you as a personal thing that I haven't shared with anyone, that the problem that I had, is that disabilities exist within your own mind. If I had to do it over again, I would ask more girls out, because the ones that I went out with, never saw me having a handicap.

William Zanke contracted polio in Wheeling, WV, in 1949 or 1950 when he was four years old.

I loved football, played it in grade school. Football in West Virginia was like it is today in Texas. The high school teams send scouts to the grade-school teams. I played football and I won an award, which was named after me, the Bill Zanke Achievement Award. I wore a brace, but when I played football, there were some guys who would come down and tape me for the games. Between eighth grade and high school, I had an operation, which allowed me to get rid of the brace, but locked the ankle in place. I went out for football, but just couldn't play with the ankle locked in place, and for years was sort of mildly resentful about that. I'm really thankful they did, but there was part of me that was conscious of the fact that people kept trying to fix me, and I didn't feel particularly broken. I still played the way you play around the neighborhood.

Puberty affected my social life; I started becoming self-conscious about limping, and was unclear about what impact that was going to have on dating and just success with women, or was convinced that it rendered me out of the game. In high school it was clear to me that the range of possible dates for me was somewhat limited; inside I knew it had to do with the limp.

Ted Kellogg contracted polio in Westfield, MA, in 1943 when he was five and a half years old.

If you were to look for one area of bitterness, college would be it. There was no way that I could attend college then. I wasn't quite strong enough to muscle my own wheelchair around. Electric wheelchairs were not practical for me back then, so I couldn't even get to classes. I made the best of what I had. I've been told that all polio victims are overachievers. I can certainly classify myself as that.

I started out with trying to get a job in the accounting field. Eventually I got this job at Electrolux by putting an ad in the paper saying, "Does anyone in the Springfield area hire the handicapped?" Sarcasm was in the ad. "Man in wheelchair, qualified accountant, needs work." It ended with "Put up or shut up." I got a call from the accounting supervisor at Electrolux, whose daughter is in a wheelchair with polio. That was my entree into the business world.

Carol Cox contracted polio in Philadelphia, PA, in 1946 when she was eighteen months old.

When I was ready to go into first grade, there was a public school walking distance for me. My mother went to enroll me. The public school denied my enrollment and said that I should stay at home and be taken care of by my family, have tutors come in; they had no way to accommodate anybody in my situation. I would be too disruptive in school. That wasn't an acceptable situation and they were not about to have me homebound for the rest of my life. They went to the Catholic school, and the Catholic school immediately said, "There's no problem. She can come in." I did go to a Catholic school all the way through college.

Everlene Brewer contracted polio in Virginia in 1945 when she was seven years old.

From the third grade through the eighth grade, I had a homebound teacher. At the end of the eighth grade, I was going to go to the regular high school, and my father had it arranged that all the classes would be upstairs. There were people who were going to put me on the bus, take me off the bus, and take me upstairs to all my classes. I had to go from class to class, within two bells. I had a lot more books to carry. I also had to worry about walking in a crowd of people. I never know who's going to knock me down—everybody was in a hurry and would get in trouble if they didn't get in class.

The third day of school, I went into my science class; there was nobody there but one woman. She said, "Could I help you?"

I said, "This is my science class."

"Oh," she said, "that's been moved downstairs."

I said, "It's not supposed to be."

"I can't tell you anything but stand in the hall."

I stood in the hall about thirty minutes. The principal's wife came by and I told her my dilemma. She said, "You have to take that up with the principal," and she kept going.

That night I started crying. Mama thought it was my homework. She said, "Oh, you can do that. You've been doing that for a long time," math.

She told Daddy that I was crying. Daddy came in and asked me why. I said, "I just can't do my math."

Mama says, "It has something to do more than the math."

I told her it was because of the situation I went through that day in school. Daddy and I and Mama go back up to school early the next morning. The principal says, "There's nothing I can do about it. You have to take science in the lab." Up we go to see the superintendent of the county. He says, "We can't change it. They do have to go to science downstairs. Nothing we can do."

Daddy says, "She's going to get an education. What are you going to do about it?"

Daddy had to take me to the elementary school. The teacher who taught seventh grade taught me one hour before class, one hour after class. During the day was a wonderful time for me. I learned how to do office work, talk on the phone. I could go substitute if a teacher needed to go out. I could grade papers. I became the librarian of the school because the principal's wife was retired. She taught me how to do the basics of a library.

Judith Ellen Heumann contracted polio in Brooklyn, NY, in 1949 when she was eighteen months old.

I don't think it's polio that affected my work and career; it's my disability. Because I could have had any disability at this level, it would have been treated the same way. Most people think I have a spinal cord injury.

Having a disability significantly reduced my work opportunities, and still does. The discrimination that exists against disabled people in employment is still very pervasive, and we don't have systems in place to enable someone with my level of disability to get accommodations on the job. In some other countries, you can get personal assistant services that you can use in your job and that are paid for in your home.

I succeeded because my parents really instilled in me the fact that you couldn't think about not succeeding. When I was growing up, there weren't really welfare programs. People who had polio went to work, or at least tried to go to work.

1950s

Steffano Graceffa contracted polio in Italy in 1953 or 1954 when he was nine months old.

I had a very high fever, and it was about four days. Trying to walk, they said it would take a little bit longer, probably eighteen months; never walked. My poor mother bought me a nice pair of brown shoes; I only wear once, and she give it to somebody else. My dad trying to discover all the doctors he knew. I had an uncle. He had a friend who was a doctor, specialized in children. He knew I had polio. My father, trying to help me out, every doctor he could. Somebody would tell him, "Go see such a doctor." We'd jump on a bus and go see the doctor.

I fell a lot. Where I was born, everything was cobblestones or black bricks from the lava. I used to bust my head. I had no control of myself walking on my right side.

In school, some of the children were very cruel. As a kid I never backed off. Even if I got my head broken, I had to fight. I feel bad in myself. I didn't accomplish anything in my life. At the age twenty-one, I went to the army base. I had to go for a physical, and the captain, when he saw me walking, said, "Son, you can't pass the physical," because he saw the scar on my leg. Broke my heart. I've never been happy.

I had a lot of trouble with the public school; my mother sent me to nun school. The teachers were the nuns. If I was two minutes late, I had to put my hands out and the nuns would hit them. If I screwed up on my homework, I had to kneel down for an hour on the concrete floor. If I said anything, I had to put my hands out, and a nun would hit me three times on each hand. If I backed away, there would be six times each hand. They would beat anybody up, and nobody couldn't say nothing.

My daddy had a very hot temper. If he knew they would beat me up, he'd go over there and beat them up. This thing went on and on, and finally I said, "I don't want to go to no more school."

Then I came to America. There was more compassion. If I was late, they wouldn't say nothing to me. They'd say, "Hey, try to be in time." Nobody would beat me up here in school.

I got married twenty years ago. I was afraid to have children because I would suspect they might have polio. I didn't understand there was a vaccine. Polio limited a lot of things in my life. My life has been destroyed.

Edward O'Connor contracted polio in Bronx, NY, in 1955 when he was ten years old.

You lied a lot because you couldn't tell potential employers that you had polio—you would never get hired. I only lost one job on account of it. The rest of them, I just lied about it.

Dottie Sternburg's husband contracted polio in Boston, MA, in 1955.

My husband, Lou, was thirty years old, and we had two young children at home. He thought he had the flu. In the evening we called the doctor who said that if I saw anything unusual during the night to let him know. He named about five things, and all five things happened during the night. I drove him to the hospital. That was the last time he walked.

This happened in August 1955. The vaccine came out in April, but they weren't giving it out yet to most people.

Lou was in an iron lung. When they would open up the lung, they'd bag-breathe him. They also taught him how to frog-breathe. Frog-breathing is when you take your tongue and push some air back down your lungs. Lou became very proficient at it and used it for his baths, for when he was on the bedpan.

Lou was transferred to a rocking bed. A rocking bed rocks from head to toe so many times a minute. There's a board at the bottom that holds your feet. When your feet went down, your diaphragm dropped. You rocked back and your diaphragm went back and that made you breathe. It's not as efficient as a chest respirator, a curette, or an iron lung. It was so much freer; he could roll over and the kids could rock on the bed with him. Lou used a chest respirator at night and the rocking bed during the day.

We bought a house before he came home. We added on a porch so that he could go outside. He came home in '56. We built a room for him and bath that was down a little hallway.

Our friends were unbelievable. It wasn't that they helped when he first came home; they did it for years. Lou was interesting and had such a good sense of humor, so our friends kept coming back. I'm not saying he didn't get depressed. He was furious about having polio, but he wasn't the kind that kept saying, "Why did it happen to me?" He was grateful it had happened to him and not to one of the kids. He became much more spiritual as time went on and he felt there was a purpose why this had happened.

Lou said, "I'd like to go back to school." A professor came to our house, who was the head of the psychology department and said, "We can do this. We'll do tape recordings of the lectures." Sometimes they'd even have seminars at our house. Some professors came to the house, some sent tapes. It took him a long time to get his master's degree and then he went for his Ph.D.

Margaret Barry Stevens contracted polio in Massachusetts in 1950 when she was twenty-six years old.

I had just had my fourth child, and when I woke up I had pains in my legs. My doctor said it must have been from the birth. I had pains in my legs off and on for the next month. I came down with a very severe headache and fever and was very tired. My husband was concerned, so he called the doctor and the doctor gave me a shot of morphine. He told me to get out of bed and walk around and I could do that then. The next day, when I went got up to go to the bathroom, my right knee buckled and I ended up on the floor. I was 26 years old, and I had four little boys.

I know how I contracted polio. The polio virus had entered the ether canisters in 1950. In those days, when you were having your babies, they gave you ether. When I woke up from having my son, I had the pains in my legs.

In the hospital, I didn't have any visitors. Even my father didn't come. They didn't even come see me when I was home. Everyone was so fearful of polio at that time. My brother-in-law told my husband to get rid of me. That was hurtful. I ended up at a state hospital, and it scared me to death.

It was like a huge dormitory. There must have been 40 beds. I never spoke to a doctor. There must have been a nurse or an orderly that took me to the room where they bake you. They put on the heat lamps so you can have passive exercises. I was parked right next to somebody in an iron lung. No one said, "This is the prognosis. This is what we're gonna do for you." I was a non-person.

One Sunday morning this cleaning woman said to me as she was mopping under the bed, "Honey, you don't need to stay here." She must have known I was miserable. I said, "Really?" That afternoon, my husband came to see me. I said, "You get me out of here." We drove home, and I never looked back.

Emily Donahue contracted polio in Ithaca, NY, in 1953 when she was seven years old.

I had spine surgery for scoliosis, and I went home with my cast on. I was really apart from everybody in my class. I would go every once in a while to a party. I'd dance with somebody, and they'd say, "Well, this is fun, dancing with this person with armor on." My mother's friend, who was a nurse, voiced a concern to me that with a cast on, I was probably never going to have much of a figure. I was not only going to be kind of skewed, but she doubted I'd ever have any breasts. She even went to the point of giving me exercises to do. When I was ready to go into eleventh grade, there was a brand-new school. I remember it was quite uncomfortable to sit, partly because the fusion had fused my pelvic bones, and I was still healing. The pressure was on and I really had to do well. My peers were all professors' children. I really separated myself from them. I just didn't feel that I could hold up my end of the competition. I made very close friends with somebody who was just a normal person—she was a cheerleader, a color guard in the band and beautiful. It was the physical side of her that I couldn't even compete with because she was so gorgeous and I was so twisted and awful-looking. I was out of my cast by then, and my body was so ugly. She liked me even though I was who I was. We remained friends through high school.

I went to Cornell. I fell in love, and I became an anorexic. The anorexia could almost have been predicted because I was beginning to see some flaws in my cerebral power. I was very nervous that I was not going to satisfy what I thought my father's standards were. Both my brother and sister had gone off wildly, so I felt a huge pressure to hold up that end. My father would tell me I was a beautiful young woman, but I didn't believe him. All I believed was that I needed to do really well in school. My boyfriend would tell me that I was beautiful, but I didn't believe him either. I was terrified of the way I looked.

The upshot of that was a complete discarding of my physical self. I didn't have to think about my body. I could focus on my academics. I told my boyfriend I couldn't see him anymore. I dismissed everybody from my life. I focused only on my studies, and I didn't eat anything. I weighed 77 pounds when I was going through this. Nobody knew what to do about anorexia in 1963.

The real crisis came when I was preparing to write my exams for my junior year. I only wrote gibberish. They weren't even words. It happened three times. I wrote for a page, and then I looked back to be sure it was okay and it wasn't. I went to the professor and said, "There seems to be some problem here." I can imagine that the professor sort of went, "Oh, that's okay. Just don't die right here in my classroom. You can take it anytime. Don't worry." I did make the courses up, but it was devastating.

I called this doctor and told him what had happened. He said, "Yeah, well, what did you expect? I knew that was going to happen." He was not very helpful, but he at least acknowledged that it was part of what was wrong with me.

I was forced to go to a psychiatrist. My mother put me in the hospital. I got out after I ate a certain amount, and I went back to school. I ate enough to get healthy somewhat, and sublimated all of the head things that were going on for years.

When I left the hospital when I had polio, I know that everybody in my family, particularly my parents, were absolutely overjoyed. They couldn't believe that I'd been able to defeat this thing. I felt singled out and handled very carefully.

When my spine fell down, the doctor said to me, "You have two options. You can either have it fixed or you cannot have it fixed. One of the reasons to have it fixed is that if you don't, you'll have a great deal of arthritis in your spine because it will be curved so badly. You'll have a big hump on your back. You won't be able to have any children." I said to myself, "That would be bad, because I'd really like to get married and have children, be a wife and mother." I went ahead with all of that.

Peggy Alford contracted polio in San Diego, CA, in 1953 when she was eighteen months old.

I remember being teased so much out on the playground. I would go home crying. That kind of thing taught me two things. It taught me to move on and realize my own self-worth. My mother was very key in that, telling me to ignore that and telling me how great I was. My parents always instilled very positive ideas into my head about me and my abilities. Then secondly, it taught me to be very empathetic towards others with handicaps. When people are in wheelchairs and children want to go inquire about them, their parents yank them away. Children learn that people with disabilities are people you need to stay away from. If you let them climb in their lap or ask them what happened, people with disabilities never mind that. They'd rather talk about it. That's where children can learn very young to respect them and realize they're people; they just operate differently.

Norma Meehan contracted polio in New Bedford, MA, in 1955 when she was four years old.

One boy hated my family. He came up behind me and pushed me down, and I had a split lip. Sister Pauline, the principal, brought me to each classroom and said, "I want to know who did this. Everyone has to stay after school until I find out." Someone told who it was. His punishment was to stay in for recess and sit next to me. He had to do homework that the nun gave him. She gave me artwork to do. She went out to the playground to check on the children. He went out the window, on the playground. The sister came in. "Where is he?"

I said, "He went out the window."

She went out and got him. She was pulling him by his ear. Once my lip healed, then I could go back out on the playground, and he could, too.

Fourth grade, there was a lay teacher, Mrs. Williams. She was eventually fired. She didn't feel that girls should have much education. She felt especially I should not be educated. I was bored in her class; I'd daydream. Or she'd do it real fast; I couldn't write down the homework assignment fast enough. I'd say, "I didn't understand. Could you tell me the homework assignment?"

She said, "There's no homework."

I'd do what I could, and then it's not all done, she'd keep me after. She was going around town with a petition for people to sign to have me institutionalized. My mother found out about it. My mother just told her off, and then put me in public school. Public school, I was sort of popular and won a contest. As the children got taller than me and developed better than me, I wasn't popular anymore, and I was teased a lot. I tried to be invisible as much as possible. They'd make fun of the sound of my brace because it squeaked a little bit.

Ann Lee Hussey contracted polio in North Berwick, ME, in 1955 when she was seventeen months old.

Kindergarten was the first time that I began to realize that I was different than other children. Children can be cruel. They can also be your best buddies, and I had a little bit of both. Some children would mimic my stride. I can remember elementary school; we had a couple of flights of stairs that we would have to climb. I could do it, but I certainly couldn't do it as fast as some of the others. We had a wonderful janitor—Mr. Clark—would carry me up the stairs, to save my energy for walking around and going outside. I have fond memories of people helping like that.

Polio did affect my not having children. We didn't want to not have children. I was pregnant, then had a miscarriage. Michael was concerned about pregnancy and taking a toll on me physically. We never pursued finding out if we had fertility problems. I never got pregnant again. I'm very blessed with some wonderful nieces and nephews, so I've filled my life with that.

Vince Huegel contracted polio in Iowa in 1954 when he was six years old.

When I got sick, I couldn't walk any more. My parents decided to take me in to the local hospital and while they were driving there they were talking to each other. They said, "Should we take him up on the elevator?" Being a farm boy, the only elevator that I knew would move grain. That really scared me because I didn't know about an elevator in the hospital. I thought they were going to take me up on one of those elevators that moved grain.

The hospital was my home away from home. It was always a busy place. The time went by fast. I was there for three months, but not really did it ever seem long to me.

I had 10 brothers and sisters, and I just kind of worked myself into the regular family schedule. They gave my dad some exercises to do with me. I had a special corner in the house where they made some pulley system where I could eat easier, to raise my arms up and down with that. I became quite independent and did things for myself.

After college I had several interviews and really didn't get anywhere doing that. Then came back home and there was a local job that I took, and that worked out fine. Sometime after I had that job, I looked for another job, and I really had trouble getting any job offers. I really think that the fact that I had polio and somebody looking at me, I didn't show as well as someone else might have.

Mary Lee Vance contracted polio in Korea in 1959 when she was two years old.

I was in the United States about the age of four. I was adopted by a Midwest family in Wisconsin. My father is a retired osteopathic physician; my mother is a retired musician. I grew up in a small community in the southern part of Wisconsin. My adoptive sister and I grew up being the only non-whites in this area. She is part Korean and part Caucasian.

I was the only kid with a real physical disability, clearly different from other children both physically in terms of race as well as with the brace. I was wearing one brace at the time. Because I was the child of the doctor in the community, who's well respected and a church-going community member, my life was, overall, pretty painless and uneventful because most people accepted me as being the doc's daughter and being a member of the community.

The differences lay with the school classmates because they did not necessarily understand or respect who my adoptive parents were. On occasion I would be prone to having insults, torments, name-callings and different kinds of stunts being acted out. I basically tried to ignore it as much as I could, and, fortunately, I feel I've been more or less unaffected by it. I just have shrugged it off and said, "That's part of life." One grows up, and everybody gets picked on in some manner, whether you're fat, short, tall, or skinny. In my case I was physically different from everyone else, and that was the reason why I got picked on.

1960s AND AFTER

Justine Guckin contracted polio in Newington, CT, in 1969 when she was two years old.

Pregnancy was hard. When I was pregnant with my daughter, I weighed almost 185 pounds, and I'm only five feet. When it came time to give birth, we found out that the place where they took the piece of my hip bone out to put into my polio leg, that's where her head went, instead of into the birth canal. They had to really work to get her out. I was in labor for more than twenty-four hours.

It was hard giving birth because my legs were uneven, so it's not like you can have some obstetric nurse hold your leg up because it's like, "Whoa, that's my little leg. You've got to be really careful of that." I couldn't leave my brace on because it was in the way. My son came out okay, thank God, he knew where to go, and he was quick.

Aimee Donohue contracted polio in China in the 1990s when she was an infant. She was adopted by American parents.

I am nine-years-old. I got polio when I was a baby. Polio made it so that sometimes I don't use the muscles that I need to so I use other ones. Sometimes we have a talk in the classroom with my physical therapist about what it was like. When other kids ask me questions I say "it just happens" and "I got it when I was a baby." I have to use braces. They support you a lot. I want other kids to know that I am a regular person. I am not an animal and it is okay to ask questions, but to not talk about it behind my back.

Jean Donohue is the adoptive mother of Aimee Donohue who contracted polio as an infant in China.

Aimee was six months old when we adopted her. We didn't know that there was any problem initially. When we were in China adopting, a lot of the older women would look at me and point to her legs and hold her legs. It wasn't until we got back here that we realized that something was wrong.

We noticed that she wasn't moving her legs very much. We weren't sure if it was just from being in the orphanage in a crib that her muscles were weak. We were sent to a neurologist, who immediately sent us to the hospital for an inpatient stay. They did a number of tests on her, and it took a while to actually come up with a diagnosis. We found out she had polio during the first month she was home with us.

The doctors told us that she probably wouldn't walk and would be in a wheelchair, but she surprised us all. She is very determined and she would crawl using her arms, and then eventually was able to pull herself to standing and at about eighteen months old she was walking.

Last year was a very difficult year for her. I think she reached an age where she was developing a maturity to know that she couldn't do everything that the other kids did. She used to love to play soccer and she just couldn't do it anymore, partially because the team is getting more competitive. Her doctors recommended that she didn't do that much in terms of exerting her legs. She went through another round of serial casting. It was done at a teaching hospital where the doctor was often explaining things to a group of students and talking about her as if she weren't in the room, which was very difficult for her.

Ewald Erilus contracted polio in Haiti in 1979 when he was three years old.

My parents came to the United States when I was about twelve years old for a better life. I haven't allowed polio to really hinder me from doing anything, other than revealing my legs. I can do a lot of the sports that I normally do without wearing any shorts, so I go about hiding it. The worst thing about the polio is feeling that you can actually break your leg doing anything. Because it looks smaller than the other, you feel like it's more fragile than the other. You're worried about it, and you don't put too much pressure on it. Then you overcompensate with the other leg, and the other one starts giving you problems.

5

THE LEGACY OF VOLUNTEERISM

The voices of polio would be incomplete without the volunteers who since the 1930s have been committed to ending polio and aiding those already stricken. From 1938 to 1962 the National Foundation for Infantile Paralysis (NFIP) and its fund-raising arm, The March of Dimes, dispatched thousands of volunteers to collect money for the campaign against polio. Other volunteers served in understaffed hospitals during the mid-century epidemics. The Salk and Sabin vaccines funded by these efforts ended the polio epidemics in the United States but did not end volunteerism. Polio survivors actively campaigned for disability rights culminating in the passage of the Americans with Disabilities Act in 1990. Polio survivors and their supporters developed post-polio support groups and the organization now known as Post-Polio Health International. Rotary International volunteers have raised significant funds to support the worldwide eradication of polio.

When polio first appeared in epidemic form in the United States, the task of trying to contain the epidemics and care for those crippled by the virus fell mainly to physicians, hospitals, and public health officials. There were, however, some precedents for the volunteer effort that characterized antipolio campaigns after 1930. For example, the National Tuberculosis Association established in 1904 included both physicians and ordinary citizens among its membership.[1] Still, the establishment of the President's Birthday Ball Commission in 1933 and the NFIP in 1938 marked a distinct departure in voluntary organizations devoted to disease eradication.

When Roosevelt purchased the resort in Warm Springs, Georgia, in 1926 to make it a center for polio rehabilitation, he had no clear idea of how to fund it. Roosevelt, with the help of his law partner Basil O'Connor, established a nonprofit foundation to run Warm Springs and raise funds. Initially the facility relied upon patient fees, support from a Patient's Aid Fund, or Roosevelt's own resources.[2] During Roosevelt's term as governor of New York, Basil O'Connor kept the facility operating even as it was losing money. To raise funds they publicized Roosevelt's own improvement at Warm Springs and the improvement

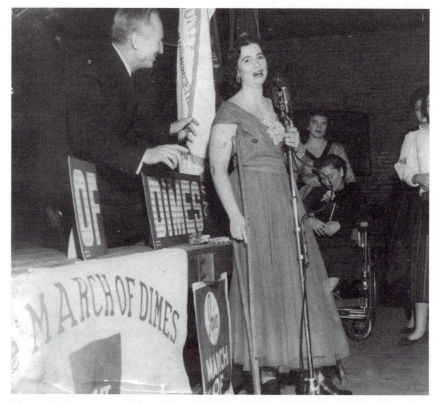

Margaret Stevens was 26 in 1950, and had just given birth to her fourth child, when she contracted polio. She is shown here speaking at a March of Dimes event in 1956. Photo courtesy of Margaret Stevens.

in many of the polio patients who were treated there. The Depression of the early thirties substantially reduced donations to the Foundation. By the time Roosevelt became president in 1933, the financial needs of Warm Springs required a new approach. A group of Roosevelt associates led by Keith Morgan came up with the plan of having a national fund-raising birthday party for the President. With Roosevelt's assent, they planned the President's Birthday Balls on January 30, 1934. There were a series of Balls across the nation that raised over one million dollars. Volunteers organized the Balls and volunteers danced and contributed their dimes and dollars.[3]

The President's Birthday Balls continued for the next few years raising fewer dollars with each succeeding campaign. By 1937 it was clear to Roosevelt's advisors that linking the President too closely to these fund-raising efforts on behalf of polio was costing them support as Roosevelt's popularity declined. In September 1937 Roosevelt announced the formation of a new national organization to fight polio. The NFIP was established in 1938 headed by Basil O'Connor.[4]

Volunteers staffed the war on polio conducted by the NFIP and the March of Dimes. Basil O'Connor, president of NFIP, was a volunteer, as were the members of the Board of Trustees and the advisory committees that guided the organization. The NFIP was organized by state and county and local organizations and took direction from the national office. Volunteers typically ran the state and county organizations. The March of Dimes, the fund-raising arm of the NFIP, was separately run and staffed on the state and local level. The NFIP volunteers oversaw the distribution of funds locally to heighten awareness about polio and to assist polio patients in paying the substantial costs of hospitalization and rehabilitation. The March of Dimes, however, recruited many more volunteers for its brief annual campaigns in December and January. In the mid-1950s the NFIP had approximately 80,000 volunteers while the March of Dimes campaigns relied on around three million. At that time, the NFIP had about 800 full-time salaried employees who managed the day-to-day operations of the organizations.[5] Between 1938 and 1962, the organization raised approximately 630 million dollars. Almost 60 percent of that provided assistance to polio patients and 11 percent went toward the research.[6]

Motives for becoming an NFIP or March of Dimes volunteer varied. Some joined because polio had struck their family or close friend, others signed up because they supported the cause. David Sills, in his study of the organization, categorized the volunteers as polio veterans, humanitarians, good citizens, and joiners. Polio veterans had come into "direct contact in some way with polio before they joined the Foundation." This group made up about 18 percent of the volunteers. Of the polio veterans, 88 percent had had polio themselves or had witnessed its affect on a family member. The other 12 percent came from the health professionals who had worked with polio patients.[7]

The humanitarians joined the organizations because they were "deeply motivated by a concern for their fellow men." As Sills observed, "the pathos of the crippled child, exhibited annually on a million posters, the promise of help to victims of a tragically disabling disease, and the hope of wiping out what is widely regarded by the American public as a major threat to the nation's children . . . attracted most Humanitarians."[8] Good citizens and joiners made up about 70 percent of the volunteer membership of the NFIP. Good citizens typically became volunteers because of "their sense of identification with their community." When polio struck they considered it their civic duty to help. Joiners were more likely to participate because they saw it as "a chance to further their own interests." Perhaps they were a local businessman or lawyer who saw participating as creating a favorable impression that would ultimately benefit their own business or firm.[9] Although their motivations for volunteering may have differed, their hard work made the NFIP and the March of Dimes successful.

The NFIP and March of Dimes volunteers came predominantly from the middle class. Many were long time residents of their communities and a majority of them had previously given time and energy to other community organizations. Sills discovered that they or their husbands were "for the most part small businessmen, lawyers, insurance agents, school superintendents, teachers, and the like—people whose status in the community is largely the result of their own efforts rather than inherited from their family's social position."[10] They had sufficient resources to donate their time, energy, and money to the polio organizations.

The March of Dimes drew most of the recruits to the cause. Sills observed that most NFIP volunteers had begun their participation as March of Dimes volunteers. The March of Dimes is often remembered for the Mother's March on Polio, which began in 1951. The Mother's March relied on the volunteer work of millions of mothers and housewives who solicited their neighbors on the chosen night. NFIP publicity urged households to turn on their porch lights to invite the marching mothers to stop for a donation. March of Dimes volunteers typically concentrated their activities into a few weeks of planning or into an hour walking their neighborhoods. Whether their commitment of time and energy was brief or extended, volunteers contributed significantly to the campaign to end polio and to help those already crippled.[11]

With the end of the polio epidemics, polio survivors, their families, and friends turned their volunteer efforts in other directions. Many polio survivors became deeply involved in the efforts to win recognition of the right of the disabled to full participation in American life. Ed Roberts and his colleagues at the University of California, Berkeley, joined in a volunteer effort to open the university to men and women with disabilities. They also created the independent living movement. Although many centers for independent living now have paid professional staffs, they are still reliant on volunteers. Other polio survivors participated in the many demonstrations across the United States that agitated for greater accessibility for individuals with disabilities. Organizations such as Disabled in Action, founded in 1970 by polio survivor Judy Heumann, ADAPT (American Disabled for Accessible Public Transit), and others pressured governments at all levels to guarantee accessibility and to pass legislation ensuring the rights of the disabled. These efforts culminated in the passage of the Americans with Disabilities Act (ADA) in 1990. Subsequently, disability activists have served as watchdogs to see that the requirements of the ADA are met.[12]

Volunteerism has also been central to the efforts of polio survivors to identify, confront, and deal with the problems of post-polio syndrome. For many years the focal point of these efforts was a volunteer named Virginia (Gini) Laurie. Named for her two older sisters who died of polio, Gini Laurie grew up sensitive to issues of disability. During the 1949 polio epidemic she became a Red Cross volunteer at the polio hospital in Cleveland. Over the years she spent many hours working with polio survivors. In 1958 she became the editor of the in-house newsletter that kept patients and survivors abreast of the hospital's activities and of survivors who had gone home. When the epidemics ended, Laurie kept this newsletter going with news of survivors as well as "self-help tips, advocacy issues, and relevant social, economic and legislative news items." In 1970 the name of the newsletter became *Rehabilitation Gazette* to reflect its broader national audience. In 1979 the *Rehabilitation Gazette* published the first letter from a polio survivor describing what would become known as post-polio syndrome. Two years later Laurie and the newsletter helped sponsor the first conference devoted to the late effects of polio. In 1983 the volunteer organization supporting the newsletter changed its name to the Gazette International Networking Institute (GINI) in recognition of Laurie's volunteer efforts. GINI continued to rely on many volunteers, but it hired its first paid executive director in 1984. Gini Laurie died in 1989, still working as a volunteer to improve the lives of polio survivors. The volunteer organization she began continues as Post-Polio Health International. It publishes a newsletter, sponsors post-polio conferences, and funds research.[13]

Beginning in the 1980s, polio survivors across the country began to create support groups to help one another deal with the physical and psychological consequences of developing new weakness, pain, and fatigue. Usually begun at the initiative of a few survivors, the support groups have reached out to all the polio survivors in their communities. Their meetings and newsletters provide information and suggestions about dealing with the problems associated with post-polio syndrome. They also provide a forum in which polio survivors can discuss what is happening to their bodies and their lives. Most of these support groups are run entirely by volunteers, although some receive assistance from Easter Seals or rehabilitation facilities.

Polio survivors have also been among the volunteers of Rotary International in its campaign to eradicate polio. Rotary International's commitment to eradicate polio began in the Philippines in 1979 when they helped begin a five-year effort to immunize some six million children against the disease. In 1985 Rotary established PolioPlus to immunize every child and pledged $120 million to the campaigns against polio. By 2005 the total contribution had risen to more than $600 million. The members of Rotary have also committed time and energy to assist the Pan American Health Organization and the World Health Organization (WHO) organize and run the immunization campaigns. Local Rotary members have been joined by American and Canadian volunteers to provide the manpower necessary to vaccinate every child in every village and hamlet.[14] A different kind of volunteer contribution came from the Bill and Melinda Gates Foundation established by the founder of Microsoft. The Gates Foundation has donated more than $1.5 billion toward the Global Children's Vaccine Fund, with many of those dollars going to support the WHO effort to eradicate polio.[15] If the WHO effort is successful, polio will join smallpox as the only diseases eliminated as threats to humans, and volunteers will once again have played a major role.

Volunteers have been central to the story of polio in the twentieth and twenty-first centuries. Polio survivors, their families, and supporters created the NFIP and the March of Dimes that raised the funds to support the scientific and medical research that developed two successful vaccines, as well as paying for many of the hospitalization and rehabilitation expenses of polio patients. Polio survivors have been important players in the decades-long effort to secure and maintain the right of individuals with disabilities to full access and participation in American life. More recently, volunteers, especially those associated with Rotary International, have kept alive the goal of eradicating polio.

THE MARCH OF DIMES

Edna Hindson contracted polio in Lake City, FL, in 1946 when she was six and a half years old.

My father had a tremendous financial burden when I had polio. In a scrapbook that I kept from that time, there is correspondence from my father to the national foundation. He's almost apologizing that he has to seek help because he was an attorney. He told me years later that he paid back the foundation, but at that time he had just so many pressures that he had to ask for help.

My mother was the local chairman for the March of Dimes and the national foundation. In my journal, there's a picture of her with Helen Hayes and Basil O'Connor. She received numerous awards for her work with the national foundation. Mother was always focused on the prevention of, with the Salk and Sabin vaccine. "Let's get money to get this disease over with."

Chester "Chet" Kennedy worked for the Department of Public Health as their art director when the polio trials were conducted in Massachusetts in 1953.

In 1953 and 1954, I became involved in the polio field trial program, working with the health educators, designing different ways that we could reach the school-age population. One of my roles was to design the information to go out to children, the communities, and physicians. I helped to design signs for school buses, and other materials that made the trials easier for them to conduct. I also helped to design the certificate. This was unique in Massachusetts. In our field trials we had the three vaccines given, and if they went through that, we gave them a button and a little card designating that they were polio pioneers. We worked with Dr. John Enders in collecting blood samples after the trials were over, and all of the children that participated in that got an additional certificate called Polio Pioneer Extraordinary. It was signed by the Governor of the Commonwealth, and presented to each one of them from the governor in a televised meeting. The kids loved it.

In Massachusetts we gave the polio vaccine to children in twenty-five communities that were selected. The criterion was that they had to have had an incidence of polio in the system before we selected them. The polio vaccine was given to almost 29,000 boys and girls in the first three grades, who participated in the trials. That was part of the nationwide program to determine whether Dr. Salk's polio vaccine would protect children from polio.

I worked with the health educators to put on presentations for the communities through parent-teacher groups and through boards of health. Health educators did community organization. We used all the media possible, which was very available at that time.

The kids had mixed emotions. There were a few of them who were still a little squeamish. The girls were better at it than the boys. We told them, "You're going to get a little prick in the arm, and it's going to be a little pain, but it'll be very brief." The big thing that sold the whole program—the health educators had done such a good job in convincing the mothers and the kids in the community that they were doing something very special.

ROTARY INTERNATIONAL

David Groner lives in Duwonjak, MI, and is a Rotarian involved in polio eradication.

I've been involved in polio eradication from the very beginning. I joined Rotary in November of 1970. The Duwonjak Rotary Club participated strongly in the fundraising in the mid 1980s, when Rotary first adopted eradicating polio as a worldwide goal. I was a Rotary district governor of southwestern Michigan, District 6360, in 1997 and 1998.

It's absolutely unacceptable that a child would be paralyzed and have their life changed for the failure to get two drops of vaccine that costs seven to nine cents to manufacture, approximately fifty to sixty cents to put on the tongues of these children. Especially in non-industrialized nations, to have this scourge when we Americans have been polio-free for decades. It's not fair to the families. It's not fair for the children. We have a responsibility as humanitarians and as people to take this easily preventable disease and distribute the vaccine to the children who do not have access to it.

In a Third World country there are not corrective surgery hospitals. There are not calipers or braces for their legs. There are not crutches for them. There are not aid societies, which assist them in everyday living opportunities, or even sheltered workshops for them to work at. These people become referred to as crawlers. If the victims are lucky, they can be on a skateboard. The life history of these people is one of deprivation, if they survive the polio at all.

In 1998, in the spring, at my district conference, my presidential representative was one Kalyan Banerjee of Bombay, India. Kalyan was a director of Rotary International. At that time one out of thirty-five children was coming down with polio in the city of Delhi. There was a massive immunization planned for December of '98, and I directed thirteen volunteers from southwestern Michigan. We joined the Rotarians and the WHO workers. On that day, our team of volunteers immunized 188,000 children in Delhi. It was a remarkable day in my life, and I have been taking volunteer teams to assist Third World countries in immunizing their children ever since.

We were only in the city probably five days. In my immunization site, which was in the ground floor of a local eight-room school, the line was four people wide, never shorter than three blocks long. The mothers were very patient to bring their children in to be immunized. The Hindi workers with me were very efficient. We did a lot of kids. We kept the vaccine cold. We had an excellent system for re-supplying our vaccine. What impressed me was the tremendous desire of the mothers to have this oral polio vaccine for their children. They weren't disorderly and pushing, but they stood their place in line. We had it posted that we would open at nine. We were ready to go at 7:15 AM, and the line had turned around the corner. I couldn't see the end of it. I was never able to see the end of it until after supper. We said we were going to close the line at five, and we closed somewhere close to ten p.m.

The following year we went to Gujarat, State of India. That would be in the north and west of India. Gujarat State had 5,000 polio cases a year. They had never gone two weeks without a polio case. We met with the Rotary District 3060 at their district conference, and we promoted a polio immunization booth. We North Americans worked that booth. I was the representative of President Carlos Reveiz. I spoke of the need to immunize.

We divided the fifty-eight people into four teams. We tried to do as much publicity with local newspapers and local governments as we could. We did everything we could to make that round of immunization a success, and we immunized, over the course of three weeks, 1.6 million children. We worked with local Rotary people, local governments, local health departments. The end result was that in the following twelve months they only had two polio cases. They went from 5,000 a year to two a year.

We worked with midwives in the slums of Bombay. Those midwives knew everybody. We worked in their clinics. When the line was getting down, you thought, "Boy, we've got everybody in this region." The midwives would talk to someone and say, "Your sister has not been here. The people on that block have not been here." Next thing you know, there'd be a hundred kids in line.

Then we went to Nigeria. We had forty in our team. We divided that forty into three groups. There were twenty-two who did the coastal area of Lagos and south. There was a team, of four women and two men that went up into the Moslem Cannel area. There was a team of four women and two men that went up into the capital, Abuja, and then three women and three men went out into the oil-drilling area to the east.

In that immunization round, we did somewhere near 38 million children—door to door. That was totally different from India. In India you set up a booth, and you expected people to come. In Nigeria, it was door-to-door, street-to-street. That was harder physically. You had to be far more cautious of keeping the vaccine under fifty degrees.

One of my teams, led by Dr. Gil O'Rourke of Jackson, Michigan, an obstetrician, immunized more than 10,000 homes in a fishing village that was up on stilts, and they walked plank to plank. The smell, the sounds, the sights, the slowness of it, was extremely challenging for that team.

I immunized the city of Apapa with the king of Apapa, who was a deacon in his Catholic church. He was a past president of his local Rotary Club. He was the landlord of all of the property in Apapa. He said to the mothers, fathers and children of Apapa, "If you don't take the vaccine, you must move. We will not have polio in our village." He marked the houses that refused the vaccine. He walked the streets with us. He gave drops.

We did islands by motorized dugout canoes. Three people had died immunizing those islands the previous year from that local Rotary Club—that was a little disconcerting. They drowned. Their boat overturned. There is an official list of people who have died immunizing children against polio.

The Nigerian experience was very positive, but it was a totally different system of immunizing than what we used in India. The infrastructure of the country, the lack of electricity, the lack of refrigeration, the lack of radio and public television, the lack of an ability to get the word out to all the small little hamlets. It's far more difficult in Nigeria than it would be in countries such as India.

Another difficult time was when Gil O'Rourke and I were immunizing. One of the families of children coming through our line were covered with maggots, both orally and rectally. When this little boy opened up his mouth, there were live flies and maggots inside his mouth. I immunized him. The family had a fungus disease of some sort, and we were able to get the family into a local hospital and get them treatment. Their treatment for a year was paid for by Jackson Rotary Club and Duwonjak Rotary Club.

Some people refuse the vaccine. In '98 in the basement of that school in Delhi, a grandfather came to me. He said, "I speak English. Would you speak to me?"

I said, "Yes, of course."

He said, "May I see it?" I put two drops of vaccine on my hand for him to see. His exact words were, "Mister, is it a trick? How can those two drops keep polio from coming to my house?" If you've never had medicine, if you've never had a vaccine, and you do not have an education where these things are discussed, it's very hard to conceive that a small dose of medicine could keep you from getting sick. The other barrier is that it's free. Being free sometimes is an obstacle because these people have never had someone care for them enough to give them anything free that was for their benefit. Finally, another factor is that we're coming as a white person from America. The grandfather went on to say to me, "May I ask you a second question?"

I said, "Of course."

"Have you given this to your children?"

"Yes, Grandfather. I have three daughters, and before I came to this place, I gave this to each of my daughters."

This man said to me, "If you had a boy grandchild, would you give it to the boy grandchild?"

I said, "Yes, of course I would. I would not want my son to have polio."

He looked me straight in the eye. He said, "I must know from you, with a straight face, looking in my eye. Is this safe for my grandchild?" That was an honest father-to-father exchange. He then said to me, "Mister, the next children in line are my grandchildren. I love them very much. I cannot have something bad happen to my grandchildren from taking this medicine. Would you give me your assurance that it's good for a grandfather to give to these grandchildren?"

I assured him; he stood right next to me, and he watched me put the drops on probably ten children. When it was finished he said to me, "Would you pray to your God who made this, that it would work for my children?"

"Yes, of course." When I said enough of this prayer, he got on his knees and he took his handkerchief and wiped my shoes. I sat on my chair and cried. He hugged me and left.

Terry Youlton is a Rotarian from Ridgetown, Ontario, Canada.

I've been a Rotarian for forty-two years. Dave Groner and I sat side by side through our trainings to be district governors. When Dave got involved in polio and going to do NIDs in India first, and then switching to Nigeria and Niger after that, I got involved with him. NID is a National Immunization Day. It started off where every child five years and under was invited to get two drops of polio vaccine on their tongue, but it was kind of a voluntary thing. They were invited to come, and everyone thought that all of the children were coming on that day to get this free vaccine. However, they found out afterwards that there were many of them hidden in the cracks that never wanted to come out, so now it's National Immunization Days. It's extended so that the first day the people are invited to come out, and then you spend the next three days going house to house, ferreting out the children who did not come on the first day.

Some children didn't come due to fear of the vaccine because this is the Sabin vaccine, the live polio vaccine. There is the occasional polio case that results from the vaccine itself.

This inoculation in places where the wild polio virus is still there, is not a once-a-year thing; it's as much as six times a year. Children who were born five years ago have been inoculated twenty-five times. Some of these parents are just absolutely sick of giving their children, time after time, two drops of polio vaccine on their tongue. Doctors say that one drop is sufficient to inoculate a child. If the child has got chronic diarrhea, then this vaccine goes right through their body, and they do not get any good of it at all. Chronic diarrhea is rampant in the same areas as polio is. The immunization in your system builds up after four or five inoculations. We don't inoculate children over five years old because they have already built up their own immune system against polio. We target children under five because 99 percent of polio cases are in children under five, and 85 percent of polio cases are in children under two. Unfortunately, a good chunk of children who get polio when they're very young die.

The people who have lost the use of both legs become crawlers. You see them crawling along the ground, mostly begging, or on some kind of a skateboard, so they can propel themselves with their hands. You see them right out in the midst of traffic, in four- and five-lane highways, wherever there's a stoplight, going from car to car, begging.

Some polio victims had their limbs that were paralyzed actually amputated because then they could put a prosthesis on and walk using the upper-limb muscles, where they couldn't walk with this piece of paralyzed flesh hanging from their knee down.

Doctors developed this Jaipur Limb made out of polyethylene pipe, molded to fit the stump of the leg, and it has a flexible rubber foot on it. The cost of that prosthesis is $35 U.S. Then they graduated into braces. They call them calipers. These are a set of braces, either for upper or lower legs that they use for polio victims. This brace costs $35 U.S. apiece.

The doctors who developed this refused to patent it because they want every possible victim in the world to use this, very cheaply and very easily. This technology has been exported to many countries in the world. The Jaipur Limb is a world-renowned prosthesis in landmine countries.

They realized that everybody couldn't come to Jaipur for getting these limbs and getting these braces, so they developed teams of a doctor and technicians who could pack up equipment and take it out to a city or town and set up a camp for a week. They would manufacture limbs and measure up braces, and custom make them to fit the victims right on the spot.

The Jaipur Limb Camps handle about 1500 victims in that weeklong period. We would make and donate to these people, between five and six hundred Jaipur Limbs or braces, some crutches. Anyone who has to stay overnight to have this limb made for them, they get a free blanket as well. They get all their food that they need for as long as they're there, and sometimes they even get a health certificate that would give them discounted travel throughout India.

Everything is paid for by Rotary. The camp that we did at Dhanbad gave out 547 limbs or braces, handled 1500-plus people, fed them, and the total cost was $29,700. The camp that we're setting up in Moradabad for November this year is costing Rotary $30,700. Our Rotary Club has sponsored two camps.

We hear, "Why are you doing all of this work for potential victims, and to stop polio from happening? Why don't you do something about the people who have polio?" I suggested to a Rotary Club that they consider having a Jaipur Limb Camp. The incoming district governor gave me the indication that he was interested. He is actually running things over there, and I'm doing the financing from over here. We are using all of the information that was collected on the first camp in Dhanbhad. That's what the Moradabad Rotary are using as their blueprint for putting this second camp on.

These 1,500 victims that come in the camp doors all are evaluated by a medical doctor, and he decides who we can help. The crawlers' limbs have atrophied so badly that they cannot be helped.

A lot of polio victims become an albatross around the neck of their parents and pull down the entire family because they cannot fend for themselves.

I led a team of young businesspeople from Detroit to Pakistan back in 1980, and there were lots of polio victims. I talked to a government official and asked, "Why didn't Pakistan at that time," 1980, "have penicillin? Why did they not use the Salk vaccine for polio?"

The guy looked at me and said, "Why? We can't feed the children that do live. Why do we want to keep any more alive?"

We have polio cornered down to just a few little parts of the world. If we don't finish it off now, it will be a major epidemic in the world again. It just spreads that fast. Nigeria stopped inoculating for the better part of a year, at least the northern states of Nigeria did. In that time period, a strain of wild polio virus re-infected six other countries around Nigeria.

Worldwide eradication is feasible. They have talked the kings in northern Nigeria into accepting the vaccines again, providing they come from Indonesia. Muslims were under the impression that the vaccine from other facilities or other manufacturers was being contaminated by something that was going to sterilize their men or women. They would only accept the vaccine that was being manufactured by a Muslim facility, and the only one is in Indonesia.

We take the money out of our own pockets to make these trips. Rotary doesn't pay one cent. The benefit goes back in your heart.

Ann Lee Hussey contracted polio in North Berwick, ME, in 1955 when she was seventeen months old.

My husband has been in Rotary for eighteen years, and I never really gave it much thought. I just participated when asked to. One day a friend of ours said, "I'm going to India to participate in National Immunization Days there, to vaccinate against polio. Would you like to come along?" I went to India on this trip with a group of Rotarians. I was still not a Rotarian at the time. Since that time, I have traveled twice more to India to participate in the immunization days there.

India was quite an eye-opener because as I was growing up, I saw a few people who had had polio. There were others in my town, older people. I never saw it in young children, and I never saw it to the degree that I saw it in India. I can remember walking down the streets of India and seeing people crawling. They would be on these little mats like mechanics use to slide under cars, and that was their mode of transportation because they were unable to walk.

I took tons of photographs of India and the people. I remember going through the photos, and noticing just by chance I had taken this picture of a crowd, and there in the foreground was this young man who was bent over, and he was walking on all fours. He had shoes on his hands and feet. Everywhere you turned in India, you would see someone who had been crippled, and it was due to polio. It was a very moving experience for me, knowing that it was possible for them not to have had polio if they'd only been vaccinated. It just made me that more supportive of the program. I was just eager to do what I could to help out.

On my first trip to India, we were visiting a rehab center where they were making some prosthetics for people and also fitting young people to braces, crutches and wheelchairs. There was this one young, beautiful, little girl. She was sitting on the bench. I looked down at her legs, and she had the same shape right leg that I did. I looked back up, and she was staring at me with this beautiful smile on her face. It just brought me to tears because it reminded me of my vulnerability when I was her age.

My biggest thing I could say is, "Yeah, it's too bad I had polio, but I'm so glad that I was in the United States when I had it," because I was given medical attention early. People in India don't necessarily see a doctor. It could be years after they've come down with polio before they're even evaluated. I've been to hospitals there and seen children having reconstructive surgery. They could be nine, thirteen, twenty-one before they're actually having any of their first surgery.

I'm a huge fan of Rotary International. It's probably one of the best-kept secrets in the world. I don't think the general public realizes how much Rotary does for so many worldwide. I think eradication is possible. It's going to take longer than we all expected initially, and the problem is going to be in Africa. We need the governments to just let the vaccinations happen.

I'm very proud to say I've been a part of, but more than proud, I'm just so happy that I've been able to help.

Joseph Serra, M.D., is an orthopedic surgeon who has operated on polio survivors in Malawi, Africa.

I'm a member of the Rotary Club of Stockton in California, and I had read about a project that was going to be undertaken in the country of Malawi back in 1980. They were selecting eight orthopedic surgeons, four of us from the United States and the other four from other countries throughout the world. We were to go to the country to actually do surgery on polio victims, primarily crawlers, people who were paralyzed as a result of polio and were unable to stand upright and walk.

The first time I went for six weeks. I was impressed with the beauty of the country of Malawi and the kind and gentle people that I met. I had no idea what to expect at first, and I was very surprised to see that the hospital where we were going to do most of the work was fairly recent. The country of Malawi had been a British colony named Nyasaland until they became independent, so there was a great deal of British influence. Many of the physicians that were in Malawi were from the U.K., including our medical director, who, he and his wife, were both family practitioners from England and they were going to be there the full two years of the project as medical director and coordinators for this project. I was impressed with the fact that there was a team in place, that the hospital was quite adequate, and that I was received very graciously by the people of Malawi.

There was an estimated 25,000 crawlers in Malawi. That was out of a population of around 8 million people. They certainly were very sad individuals. They had a nickname for them that literally meant that they didn't even exist because it was difficult for them to get an education because this physically crawling back and forth to school was difficult.

Many of them would gravitate to the cities because it was safer than living in the bush because they could be dragged away by animals. Some were killed by snakes because they were crawling on the ground and would be struck in the head or neck. Crawlers were the beggars in the cities, and many of them sat outside doors, banks, and bus stations and sold souvenirs to people. There's crawlers in most of the developing world—India, the Philippines and places where they couldn't be treated.

The attitude was one of "We know they're there. We can't do anything to help them." There were no orthopedic surgeons in the country. There were only about 150 doctors for that many people, which meant about one doctor per every 50,000 people. Medical care was quite basic. Funds for providing medical care to the population were about five dollars per person per year.

None of these crawlers had really been treated because there were no orthopedists there to do the work. Those that were doing orthopedic-type surgery were primarily treating trauma, broken bones. They didn't have the expertise to do anything with the crawlers. Those of us that had the training in orthopedic surgery knew we could straighten their legs and lengthen their tendons so that we could get them into braces and get them upright and walking. That was our goal, to operate on crawlers, do as many as we could, do the simplest procedures that we could do for the beginning cases, the first several months, and get as many on their feet and get them going back to their villages where other crawlers could see the results and would then come in to see our team.

We did over 2,400 operations, but some of the patients would have to have two or three procedures before we had their leg fairly straight. Many of the patients that we saw didn't require surgery, just braces or wheelchairs to get them off the ground. We had an excellent team. We had five physical therapists that were with us full time, three from the Netherlands, one from the U.K., and one from Malawi, that were able to not only do rehab, but also identify polio cases that were good candidates for our surgery. It was important to us that our patients be screened, that we select the ones that we could help the best. They had to have good strong backs and good upper arms so that once we had their legs straight, they could put on their braces and stand up and walk. These patients were selected quite carefully and extremely well by our team of physical therapists and physicians.

I had such a great experience when I went there the first time that I went back in 1983 for the second tour, and then again in 1986. The project was actually extended to three years because we were doing so well and we still had some funds left out of the initial grant. Some Rotary districts and clubs in various parts of the world gave us more funds to keep going.

WORLD HEALTH ORGANIZATION (WHO)

Bruce Alyward, M.D., directs the polio eradication effort at the WHO.

I worked in Uganda, at the end of the war there, as part of my medical training. While there—I went there with a measles project—I saw a lot of polio.

A man who had contracted polio some years earlier was living in an iron lung. During the day, it was okay. He could breathe on his own, but at night the family members had to stay up and pump to keep this iron lung going. I've maintained this great interest in immunization. Years later, I did a Master's in public health at Johns Hopkins, and there was a chance to intern at the WHO. I spent a couple of months in Geneva with them, and there were great opportunities with this new polio program that was coming up. I spent the next 14 years in the program. I've worked dozens of countries, helping set up the programs, in five of our regional programs, and I've run the program here in Geneva. Since 1998 I've been the head of the overall program.

It definitely is possible to eradicate this disease. Whether the world will put all the will behind it to achieve it, I increasingly think so. G8 Summits, APEC Summits, heads of state are all part of this program. Political implications of failure are very great. It's getting to the point where I believe there would have to be a major technical failing for it to fail, or the world to just run out of the will to put the money into it.

6

THE IMPACT ON DISABILITY RIGHTS IN AMERICA

Polio survivors began as early as the 1930s to push for recognition of the rights of individuals with disabilities. They began to rethink the problem of disability, recognizing that the problem was not so much in the individual with the impairment, as in the culture's outmoded conceptions about people with disabilities and in society's failure to provide equal access and opportunity regardless of one's impairment. And just as African Americans in the fifties and sixties claimed the political and civil rights so long denied them, many polio survivors agitated for the rights of the disabled.

President Franklin D. Roosevelt was a role model for many polio survivors. If he could overcome polio to become president, then anything was possible for those who had had polio.[1] At least that was the message that Roosevelt seemed to convey and that many polio survivors wanted to believe. However, Roosevelt's legacy for polio survivors and other Americans with disabilities was more complicated and ambiguous than his mythic image. In order to have a political career, Roosevelt largely concealed the extent of his disability with the help of a complicit press. The historian John Duffy concluded that while Roosevelt certainly demonstrated that polio was not necessarily a barrier to success, he did little during his terms in office to enable "disabled people to overcome the physical barriers and consequently the social prejudices they faced."[2] More recently, Amy Fairchild argued that even among polio survivors Roosevelt's legacy is mixed. While he served as "hero and role model" to polio survivors in the thirties and forties, those who had polio in the post–World War II era began to shake off the influence of the mythic Roosevelt.[3] The sociologist and polio survivor Irving Kenneth Zola wrote that "few of us can control, manipulate, and overcome our environment the way FDR did." He recognized that the mythic Roosevelt set a potential trap for ordinary men and women with disabilities: "if a Franklin Delano Roosevelt . . . could overcome [his] handicaps so could and should all the disabled. And if we fail, it is our problem, our personality defect, our weakness."[4] Polio survivors like Zola who came of age during the civil rights movement began to realize that society created the barriers people with disabilities faced. If society was responsible for the barriers, then it was society's responsibility to remove them. And with that insight the disability rights movement was born.

Ironically, one of the first efforts of polio survivors to advocate for greater rights for individuals with disabilities came during Roosevelt's first term as president. The League of the Physically Handicapped was established in New York City in 1935 by a group of men and women, many of them polio survivors, who had encountered discrimination when applying for jobs. The League had its origin in the discriminatory policies of federal relief programs designed to aid unemployed workers. The Works Progress Administration (WPA), a major relief program for unemployed workers and part of Roosevelt's New Deal, declared the handicapped to be unemployable and thus not eligible for assistance.[5] Several disabled young adults challenged their exclusion from jobs under the WPA program. On May 29, 1935, six of them went to see the director of the New York office of the Emergency Relief Bureau to "demand an end to disability-based discrimination in work relief." When he refused to see them, they began a sit-in that lasted until June 6. However, the sit-in and the outside protest that accompanied it produced few results. After the sit-in ended several of the protesters established the League of the Physically Handicapped to continue agitating for equal access.[6] The historian Paul Longmore notes that although the League of the Physically Handicapped "failed to redirect federal policies, it continued to oppose job discrimination in New York City" and advocated opening "the public sector to workers with disabilities." Ultimately their efforts pushed the WPA in New York to hire approximately fifteen hundred men and women with disabilities, some of whom would eventually move into "civil-service careers."[7] In spite of the League's limited success, their activities marked a new activist approach to addressing the problems of individuals with disabilities. As Longmore writes, the League "concentrated on discrimination rather than diagnosis," and "their activism sought to alter public understanding of disability, shifting the focus from coping with impairment to managing identity, from experiencing polio to engaging in politics."[8]

In the forties and fifties, the determination of so many polio survivors to enter the mainstream of American life had the greatest impact on the rights of individuals with disabilities. When the polio epidemics were at their worst, virtually everyone in the United States knew someone who had polio. The presence of someone in the neighborhood, in school, or in the workplace who relied on braces, crutches, or a wheelchair for mobility became commonplace. Their very success in school, in raising a family, and in earning a living demonstrated over and over again that a physical impairment was not necessarily a barrier to succeeding at the ordinary tasks and responsibilities of life in America. As many of the oral histories demonstrate, in these decades it was usually the polio survivor who had to make the accommodations, who had to figure out ways to surmount the barriers that so often barred access to school and work. American society was not yet ready to acknowledge equal access as a right guaranteed to all Americans regardless of their impairments.

The next step would be taken in the 1960s after the University of California, Berkeley, admitted Ed Roberts who was severely paralyzed by polio at age fourteen. As he recovered his strength in the years that followed, Roberts eventually returned to school in a wheelchair, although he still relied on an iron lung for part of the day. After his parents fought to have the physical education and driver education requirements waived, Roberts graduated from high school and began attending nearby San Mateo Community College. Two years later, his academic advisor urged him to apply to Berkeley because it had a good program in his chosen field of political science. Two obstacles appeared. The California Department of Rehabilitation refused to pay his tuition on the grounds that he would never be able to work. After negative publicity in the papers, the department reversed its decision. The second obstacle was the university itself, which refused to admit him saying, in the words of one dean, "We've tried cripples before and it didn't work." Parts of the campus were inaccessible to wheelchair users and there was no accessible housing on campus. Roberts, however, soon found an advocate in Dr. Henry Bruyn, the director of student health services, who arranged for Roberts to move his iron lung into the university's Cowell Hospital. With assistants to push his wheelchair, and occasionally lift him into buildings, Roberts lived on campus and attended classes.[9] After newspapers printed articles describing Roberts's experience at Berkeley, other severely disabled young men and women applied for admission. By 1967 there were twelve of them living in the university hospital and calling themselves the "Rolling Quads." The students living in Cowell Hospital connected their struggles to achieve an education and an independent life to the civil rights struggles taking place across the nation. They persuaded the university to create a program to assist students with disabilities and to create accessible housing and they convinced Berkeley to install curb cuts so individuals in wheelchairs could more easily move around the city. In 1970 Roberts and his associates received a U.S. government grant to establish the Physically Disabled Students Program (PDSP) at Berkeley. The program helped students with disabilities find housing and attendants as well as deal with the university bureaucracy. Their philosophy was more radical than the assistance that the PDSP provided. "Roberts redefined independence as the control a disabled person had over his life. Independence was measured not by the tasks one could perform without assistance but by the quality of one's life with help."[10]

The success of the PDSP at Berkeley led Roberts and his coworkers to establish a similar program for nonstudents. The first Center for Independent Living (CIL) was created in the spring of 1972 in Berkeley. The CIL "would be run by disabled people; approach their problems as social issues; work with a broad range of disabilities; and make integration into the community its chief goal." Roberts became director of the CIL in 1974. He left the organization in 1975 when Governor Jerry Brown appointed him director of the California Department of Rehabilitation, the same organization that had once declared him unemployable. The success of the Berkeley Center for

Independent Living soon served as a model for similar centers across the country.[11]

Ed Roberts was not the only polio survivor to be moved to action by the example of the civil rights movement. Struck with polio when only eighteen months old, Judy Heumann was left a quadriplegic. After graduating from high school, Heumann attended Long Island University where she fought to make the university more accessible and organized other disabled students to push for the needed changes. When she finished the program she was denied her teaching certificate because she could not pass the medical exam. She sued the Board of Education and took her case to the newspapers. The board settled out of court and Heumann received her certification. In 1970, when she was twenty-two, Heumann established a disability rights group, Disabled in Action (DIA). Heumann's DIA was more overtly political than the CIL and engaged in frequent political protests against the treatment accorded individuals with disabilities. In 1971 Heumann went to California to work with Ed Roberts and the CIL in Berkeley and from 1975 to 1982 she served as the deputy director of the CIL. Like Roberts, Heumann would later serve in government as Assistant Secretary of Education in the Clinton administration.[12]

The stirrings of protest among individuals with disabilities occurred not only in major cities like Berkeley and New York, but even in such places as the conservative Lehigh Valley of eastern Pennsylvania. In 1973, Carl Odhner, a polio survivor, organized a protest against plans to renovate the major downtown street without curb cuts. The demonstration was effective and when the street was reconstructed it included curb cuts. Odhner then organized Operation Overcome to continue advocating for the rights of men and women with disabilities. In 1990 Odhner and his associates established the Lehigh Valley Center for Independent Living on the model of the Berkeley CIL.[13]

Ron Mace, who had polio in 1950 at the age of nine, took a somewhat different approach to improving the lives of individuals with disabilities. Mace attended North Carolina State University where he often had to be carried into inaccessible buildings. A 1966 graduate in architecture from the university's School of Design, Mace became a practicing architect before getting involved in developing the first building code in the United States to incorporate principles of accessibility. The code became law in North Carolina in 1973 and would serve as a model statute for other states. He was later involved in drafting and building support for mandated accessibility in federally funded programs and for the 1990 Americans with Disabilities Act (ADA). After working in conventional architecture for several years, Mace focused his practice on what he called "universal design." Universal design is designing architecture and interior furnishings so that they are accessible and usable by individuals with a wide range of abilities and disabilities. Mace's work was an important adjunct to activists like Roberts and Heumann. When establishments and institutions protested that accessibility was too costly, Mace and his colleagues could demonstrate how easily and inexpensively buildings could be made accessible to all.[14]

Like Ron Mace, Hugh Gallagher, who had polio in 1952 while a student at Haverford College, worked behind the scenes helping to draft legislation that would make the nation more accessible to individuals with disabilities. While working on the United States Senate staff he pressured institutions such as the Library of Congress to make their facilities accessible. Gallagher also played a major role in writing the Federal Architectural Barriers Act of 1968 that required that federal buildings be accessible.[15]

Polio survivors were also active in building the political coalition that would finally secure passage of the ADA in 1990. A key figure behind the enactment of the ADA was Justin Dart, Jr. Born into a wealthy family in 1930, Dart had polio when he was eighteen. After polio he earned a bachelor's and a master's degree from the University of Houston planning to become a teacher. But like Heumann, he was not awarded a teaching certificate because he used a wheelchair. He went into business instead, building successful companies in Mexico and Japan. In the mid-sixties Dart sold his business and focused his energies on human and disability rights. Dart, a Republican most of his life, served on the Texas Governor's Committee for Persons with Disabilities, as vice chair of the National Council on Disability under Ronald Reagan, and as director of the federal Rehabilitation Services Administration. Beginning in the mid-eighties Dart traveled widely to build support for the ADA as well as lobbying individual congressmen and senators. Dart always acknowledged the many other people who helped secure passage of the ADA, but he clearly merited President George H.W. Bush's observation that Dart was "the ADA man."[16]

Polio survivors were not alone in their efforts to expand the civil rights of individuals with disabilities and to make the United States more accessible to persons with a wide range of impairments. Advocates for individuals who were blind and deaf or otherwise disabled, veterans disabled in service to their country, and parents seeking greater opportunities for their children with physical and mental impairments all contributed to the passage of state and federal laws beginning in the 1960s and continuing to the ADA in 1990. Still, it is remarkable how many polio survivors participated both locally and nationally in the long effort to recognize and protect the rights of individuals with disabilities. That effort often had its origins in their own efforts to meet the psychological, attitudinal, and physical barriers to participation in American society in the decades following World War II. But it was also part of the context of the times in which other disadvantaged groups such as women and African Americans agitated for the rights so long denied them. As a result of the work of polio survivors like Ed Roberts, Judith Heumann, Carl Odhner, Hugh Gallagher, Ron Mace, and Justin Dart the legal framework for recognizing and protecting the rights of individuals with disabilities has been established. However, the more recent attacks on the ADA and other laws and regulations mean that the work has only begun. As these oral histories reveal, polio survivors are still part of the continuing fight for disability rights.

Edna Hindson contracted polio in Lake City, FL, in 1946 when she was six and a
half years old.

I moved to Lake City, Florida in 1975. In 1976 communities were trying to do projects for the bicentennial. I called some folks and said, "Let's make our project curb cuts," because people now can't believe they didn't have curb cuts back then, but they didn't. We got the National Guard and some volunteers and started out with a small section of Lake City. We got cement donated, and we were gradually getting curb cuts around this community as our little project. We were trying to talk to different businesses about how important it was to be able to have people in wheelchairs get into a store.

I was hired in 1988 as the compliance person at a community college. I worked with physical plant. There was just so much money with a small community college, so we didn't try to do everything at once. I'd say, "Don't you think we can just do one automatic opening door this semester?" I got bids from different companies and then we'd sit down together and let them decide which company to use. We'd just try to do one project a semester. Now it just thrills me to go out to that campus, and it is the correct doorknob handles, the Braille on the—everything that they totally require now.

I developed Disability Awareness Day. We were probably the first college. Our college won twice at national levels. We had our gym set up with all the vendors of all the different equipment that people with disabilities need to know about. Where the person may want a van, but they just can't get around to try out all the different vans that have the lift on them. We would get the companies to bring in samples of wheelchairs, adaptive equipment. Anything you can think that relates to any of the disabilities as far as equipment and services, we had exhibit booths.

Judith Ellen Heumann contracted polio in Brooklyn, NY, in 1949 when she was
eighteen months old.

Having any disabled child in the family does alter the way the family moves forward because there were all these things that they had to be doing for me, which weren't typically done for other kids in other families. Things like having me going to the doctor and going to therapy.

My parents made a commitment early on that they wanted me to be able to have the same opportunities as they had thought about for me prior to becoming disabled. I learned later on in life that there was a doctor that had recommended to my parents that they place me in an institution because my disability was significant, and it would make it easier for them to take care of my brother and have future children. My parents didn't do that.

I felt uncomfortable in high school because I didn't have a motorized chair, and I wasn't strong enough to push myself, so there was an aide. The aide used to help me get from class to class. I needed help going to the bathroom, so there was somebody who would help me. That made me feel like I stuck out because I couldn't get around myself.

When I was graduating from high school, I was getting an award and was supposed to go onstage to receive the award. The night of the high school graduation, my father was about to pull my wheelchair up the stairs. The principal said that he didn't want me to go up onto the stage. I could sit in the front row, and they would come and give me the award. I told my parents that I wanted to leave. My parents insisted that I be allowed on the stage. I was so angry that I started crying.

I don't think it's polio that affected my work and career; it's my disability that affected my work and career. Because I could have had any disability at this level, it would have been treated the same way. Most people have no idea what condition I have. They think I have a spinal cord injury.

Having a disability significantly reduced my work opportunities, and still does. The discrimination that exists against disabled people in employment is still very pervasive, and we don't have systems in place to enable someone with my level of disability to get accommodations on the job. In some other countries, you can get personal assistant services that you can use in your job and that are paid for in your home.

I succeeded because my parents really instilled in me the fact that you couldn't think about not succeeding. When I was growing up, there weren't really welfare programs. People who had polio went to work, or at least tried to go to work.

I've always worked, even though it has been difficult to get jobs. When I graduated from college, I was trying to get a job as a social worker. I had applied for a position and then an interview over the phone and had a really good interview with this individual. We set up a time for me to come in and do a face-to-face interview. When I hung up, I called back because I realized I needed to tell him that I wanted to know if the place was accessible. As soon as they found out that I was in a wheelchair, they weren't interested in interviewing me anymore.

I had to go to court to get my teaching license because they denied me my teaching license because I couldn't walk. I passed the written exam; I passed the oral exam, but I was failed the medical exam, because I couldn't walk. I sued the Board of Education, got my license and then taught.

I did get to teach for three years. Then I got very heavily involved in the Disability Movement which I had started working on before I began teaching. From about 1967 on, I was very involved in the movement. Later, I went to the Berkeley Center for Independent Living and worked there. At UC Berkeley at that time, the Disability Movement was evolving, and there was a disabled students program that was becoming active. Many of the buildings were still not accessible. I was in the School of Public Health, and they had no accessible bathroom. Every time I had to go to the bathroom, I had to go to the Disabled Students Program, which was off campus. At that point I had a motorized wheelchair.

I was really one of the second-level founders for the Center for Independent Living. It started in 1972, and I came in 1973. I worked with Ed Roberts, who had polio, and another person. Until now, all of my positions have either been in disability organizations or working for the federal government in the Clinton administration or now at the World Bank on disability issues. I'm a very strong advocate on disability issues, and I'm very proud of that. Being a strong advocate in disability is different than a strong advocate in gender or in the Labor Movement or in the Civil Rights Movement or the People of Color Movement. People still don't understand the issues. They tend to try to marginalize you because they're unwilling to accept the fact that you understand issues. You have to prove you're a loyal member of the team, that you're working for the same agenda, that our issues are similar to the issues of other movements. It's very, very interesting.

John Hager contracted polio in either Richmond, VA, or Greenwich, CT, in 1973 when he was thirty-one years old.

I contracted polio in 1973 and it came at a very devastating point in my life because I was a young, upcoming corporate executive and had been notified that I was promoted and was being transferred to our New York office. My wife and I, with a baby, had bought a new house in Greenwich, Connecticut, and we were in the process of selling the house we had in Richmond, Virginia. Our son Jack went on a routine visit to the pediatrician and was administered the Sabin oral polio vaccine. That evening he became violently ill. Through some contact with his throwing up or the diapers, I became exposed to the Sabin vaccine that had been administered to the child. I was called a "contact case," and acquired polio from the live virus in that vaccine.

I have not necessarily been an outspoken advocate, but have certainly participated with people with disabilities in a variety of fashions, including chairing the Disability Commission in Virginia because the four years I served as lieutenant governor, by statute was the chairman of the Disability Commission; and by working on fundraising efforts with many of the civic and charitable organizations that help people with disabilities, like Easter Seals. I received the national Easter Seals award, the Platte Award, for community service. I've done a lot with people with disabilities, but I have not directly been an advocate.

No one properly diagnosed my case. I became paralyzed from the neck down. In the emergency room, they had a myelogram. That was the state of the art in those days. They didn't have CAT scans and MRIs then. The myelogram showed a couple of discs in my back that were out of line. That had probably happened during the onset period of about ten days when I kept stumbling and falling down. Out jogging early in the morning, I fell down and knocked myself out. Somehow I had hurt my back in this painful onset period. The physicians in the emergency room saw these out-of-line discs and assumed that there was a malignant tumor that was pushing those discs out of line. They operated on my back. In addition to having a severe case of polio,

I had a major back operation. They found nothing, other than two discs that were recently dislocated. They trimmed the discs and sewed me up.

When I recovered, I was denied the work promotion. They thought maybe I'd be better off not moving to New York, that it might be difficult to get around. The culture was quite different then, and no one was ready to accept someone in a wheelchair. I had to, in essence, start all over.

I've done so many things. I've been chairman or president of thirty different organizations. I've been a lieutenant governor for four years. I was an Office of Homeland Security director for two and a half years, starting right after 9/11. Now I'm going to be Assistant Secretary of Education.

I went to Harvard Business School, and my goal in life has always been in management structure and organization. I like to get things done, and I like to be effective. I think that comes from my business school and training in engineering prior to that. Whether it's with homeland security, education, it's with whatever impacts disability in whatever fashion, I'm a great believer in the management approach, so I tend to apply it to disability like I would apply it to anything else.

Joan Headley contracted polio in Ohio in 1948 when she was fifteen months old.
In high school I went in to talk to the guidance counselor about colleges. I can remember him saying, "Well, you know, you might want to consider being a teacher or a nurse, because they need teachers and they need nurses, and no matter where your husband goes, why, you can find a job." I think that was interesting how he was framing what my career would be in perspective of what my husband might do. He did influence me to the point that I did become a teacher. 1965 was the year that the Voc Rehab Bill was enacted. It was brand new and Mary Switzer had gotten a lot of money from Congress so that people who had disabilities could go to school and get an education. Her philosophy was that if people with disabilities got an education, then they could get jobs be tax-paying citizens. I was definitely a beneficiary of that. The registrar said to me, "Because you're handicapped, we can apply to Vocational Rehabilitation and they will pay for your room and board, and tuition." It was a godsend. I can remember thinking that that's really interesting because I hadn't ever labeled myself as being handicapped or having a disability.

Later in life I ended up in St. Louis, working for Gini Laurie. When the disability rights people talk about the Independent Living Movement, they talk about the two grandmothers of the Independent Living Movement; and one was Mary Switzer and the other was Gini Laurie.

I worked with Gini Laurie to help create this organization that has certain parameters, but it's also an umbrella that we can include lots of polio survivors no matter where they are on the spectrum. That umbrella that we created subscribes to that whole larger idea about the civil rights of people and the whole idea of the independent living movement, and letting polio survivors have an opportunity to improve their life from things that they've learned from our organization, for them to learn to advocate for themselves.

There are many organizations that help polio people all across the country and all across the world. Our organization encourages polio survivors to do things locally, and do what they think needs to be done in their community, and we're there to help and advise them if they want it. We play a pivotal role in keeping all of those organizations connected.

Robert Lonardo contracted polio in Rhode Island in 1935 when he was three years old.

My twin brother was very athletic, and all the friends we hung around with were very active. I had to keep up with them, and it was a continual struggle. Even though I couldn't run, I made up for it. I had pretty good reflexes. I had agility everywhere but on my leg. I would do everything they did. I think that had a lot to do with what I wound up doing and how I looked at things. I did not consider myself to be handicapped and limited, even though it was a struggle to carry myself a certain way not to look crippled. Polio broke my heart. I really wanted to be just like everybody else. I didn't accept my disability. I didn't accept my limitations.

Fred Faye sustained a spinal cord injury in the Washington, DC, area in 1961 when he was sixteen years old.

I broke my neck in 1961 and knew virtually nothing about disability at the time. I soon discovered the world around me wasn't that accessible, and decided to try to do something about it. The biggest problem was the attitudes of able-bodied people in a society where if you saw a person with a disability at a movie or a TV show, it was almost always a very stereotyped role, the arch villain or a Tiny Tim. My first involvement in any sort of a movement came about a month after I broke my neck. I was out at Georgia Warm Springs Foundation, and I met a lot of other people in wheelchairs—mostly post-polios. I went from Warm Springs back to Washington, D.C., where I'd been born and grew up, and found every corner had a curb. There were no ramps at all. The city, in spite of having a president in a wheelchair, was inaccessible. Even in the White House, the ramps they built to accommodate FDR were taken down immediately after he was out of office.

I started a group called Opening Doors back in 1963 based on my Warm Springs experience. One of our goals was to provide peer counselors to newly disabled people in the Washington, D.C., area, and the other was to develop a list of wheelchair-accessible buildings, restaurants and hotels and theaters, of which there were very few at the time. In the early seventies, I co-founded the American Coalition of Persons with Disabilities, which was a cross-disability group. We had paraplegics, people who were blind and deaf, all members of this umbrella organization.

Now I spend a good deal of time on the Internet to do advocacy. With the keyboard and Worldwide Web, it's so easy. Forty years ago, I used the telephone and mail and newsletters. It was very difficult. For example if there was an advocacy issue before Congress, by the time the message was printed and got to the advocates around the country to congressional people, they had already taken the vote. Eventually we got bulletin boards, then e-mail, that helped, and more recently listservs. Now with cell phones you can track people down wherever they are to give them the advocacy message.

7

POST-POLIO SYNDROME

When polio survivors completed their rehabilitation many came away with the impression that their impairments would be stable over time, and that they would not become any more disabled. However, in the late 1970s and 1980s many polio survivors from the mid-century epidemics began to experience puzzling new symptoms including increased pain, fatigue, and muscle weakness. Intuitively, many suspected that these changes were related somehow to polio and to the strains and stresses of living with a disability. Many initially tried to apply the old polio rehabilitation philosophy of "use it or lose it" only to discover that their symptoms worsened.

Clearly something disturbing was happening to their bodies, but initially they found little support or information from the medical profession. Doctors attributed the symptoms to the normal problems of aging, or suggested that polio survivors consult a psychiatrist to address problems that "were all in their heads." Polio survivors knew better, and their advocacy and insistence eventually brought medical recognition and appropriate treatment strategies. Polio survivors often experienced these new problems as a second disability. In the oral histories, polio survivors discuss the difficulties they had in finding sound medical advice and effective treatment strategies, the challenges of living with new impairments, and the psychological costs of developing a second disability late in life.

Post-polio syndrome is a recent diagnosis for the late effects of polio, but the problems it describes have probably been around as long as polio. In reviewing the medical literature on the late effects of polio, Dr. David O. Wiechers discovered that the symptoms ascribed to post-polio syndrome in the 1980s and 1990s had been first described by the great French neurologist Jean Martin Charcot in 1875. Throughout the late nineteenth and twentieth centuries scattered reports and case studies appeared in the medical literature describing the emergence of new symptoms that seemed to be associated in some fashion with a previous case of polio. In the 1960s and 1970s, physicians began to conduct studies on polio survivors who were experiencing

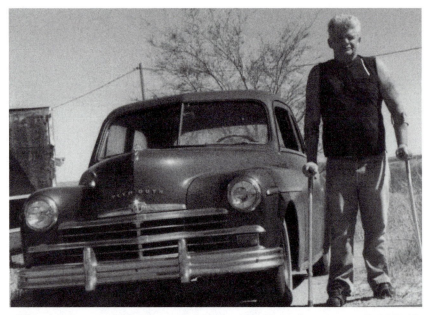

Rick Spalsbury never got any treatment after contracting polio at age two in 1945. His parents' religion did not allow medical treatment. He says they were embarrassed by his inability to walk. "They would put me in the closet when they had company." Photo courtesy of Rick Spalsbury.

new difficulties.[1] Doctors had given post-polio syndrome little attention in the decades when the polio epidemics were at their height. Virtually all medical efforts then went toward caring for and rehabilitating the new cases. After the epidemics ended, the complaints of the aging polio survivors were more visible than they had been earlier, and the many survivors from the mid-century epidemics meant that the late effects of polio affected significant numbers of men and women. In addition, the advocacy efforts of polio survivors helped doctors in the 1980s to take the problems of post-polio syndrome seriously and to develop care and treatment strategies. Where there were only scattered articles on the late effects of polio before 1970, over 450 scientific and medical articles on post-polio syndrome have been published since 1967.[2]

The *Rehabilitation Gazette* and its successors as well as the variously titled post-polio organization ably headed by Gini Laurie and Joan Headley have provided a focal point for the polio survivors' advocacy. A 1979 letter by Larry Schneider in *Rehabilitation Gazette* alerted readers to the new and disturbing problems and the inability of physicians to provide either an explanation or effective treatment. Two years later *Rehabilitation Gazette* sponsored a conference in Chicago organized by Gini Laurie to examine these puzzling developments. Over two hundred doctors, scientists, and polio survivors attended. A second conference held in St. Louis in 1983 led to the creation of the Gazette International Networking Institute (GINI) to coordinate the efforts of polio survivors and sympathetic physicians to understand the late effects of polio. GINI, which became Post-Polio Health International in 2003, has sponsored nine post-polio and independent living conferences. The organization has also continued to publish newsletters to inform polio survivors of the most recent developments and has more recently raised funds to support research on post-polio syndrome.[3] However, many polio survivors are discouraged by research efforts and believe that not enough is being done.

Post-polio syndrome often begins with little more than a hesitation in one's step, or a slight increase in pain or fatigue. These small changes may seem unremarkable to polio survivors accustomed to dealing with their long-standing impairments. But over weeks and months the changes add up. The stumbles and falls occur with distressing regularity. The pain becomes more insistent and the fatigue more noticeable. Then simple actions become impossible. The increased pain and fatigue mean more days absent from work. Something definitely has changed. Most of the physicians polio survivors consulted in the 1970s and 1980s were unable to provide either an explanation for what was happening or treatments that reduced or eliminated the symptoms. Many younger doctors had never treated a case of acute polio, let alone the late effects of polio. Some physicians explained the symptoms as the normal effects of aging, prescribed physical therapy for the weakened muscles, or, sometimes, suggested that the problems were psychological in origin.

More recently, however, the advocacy efforts of polio survivors and sympathetic physicians have increased knowledge about post-polio syndrome among both survivors and doctors. Several recent handbooks and manuals for living with post-polio syndrome have been published that have enabled polio survivors to become well informed medical consumers and they have provided physicians with the basic information they need to properly diagnose and treat the late effects of polio.[4]

The increased availability of knowledge about post-polio syndrome has significantly reduced the uncertainty and confusion that surrounded the emergence of the problems of polio survivors in the seventies and eighties. However, the late effects of polio still pose a considerable challenge to polio survivors and their families. Many polio survivors developed a healthy aversion to doctors during their long rehabilitation from the disease and have been reluctant to place themselves once again under the care of doctors, especially doctors who have little experience in working with polio patients. The decision to seek medical help did not, moreover, always bring immediate relief. Many survivors went from doctor to doctor for months or even years before gaining a satisfactory explanation of the physical changes they were experiencing and before being advised on helpful treatment. The anxiety of not knowing what was happening to their bodies only compounded the challenge of dealing with new and often debilitating symptoms.

Family members also found it difficult to deal with the emergence of the late effects of polio. Polio survivors have a well-deserved reputation for finding ways to do what they need to do in spite of their disabilities, and doing it with an upbeat outlook. Families and friends became accustomed to this polio persona and its can-do attitude. When polio survivors found they could no longer walk as far, carry as much, work as hard, or participate as fully as they always had, families often had trouble adjusting. In addition, the survivors often found it hard to convey the pain, frustration, and anxiety they were feeling. Over time many family members and others came to accept the reality of physical changes brought by post-polio syndrome, but the process was often difficult for both the survivors and those they lived and worked with.

Post-polio has come to be recognized as having certain characteristic symptoms: "new weakness, unaccustomed fatigue, muscular pain, new swallowing problems, new respiratory problems, cold intolerance, and new muscle atrophy." But as Dr. Julie Silver writes in her guide for polio survivors, "PPS [post-polio syndrome] is a diagnosis of exclusion."[5] Individuals with the above symptoms must also meet four criteria for a diagnosis of post-polio syndrome: "1. An individual must have a known history of polio; 2. The individual must have had some improvement in strength following the initial paralysis; 3. There must have been a period of stability (at least one or two decades) in which the individual had no new symptoms; 4. The individual must present with new symptoms that are consistent with PPS and not attributable to some other disease."[6] There are also cases that are more difficult to diagnose where the individual may have had an unapparent case of polio or only mild temporary paralysis.[7] Thus, even now when the typical symptoms of post-polio syndrome are better understood, securing a definite diagnosis can still sometimes be difficult.

Treatment for post-polio syndrome needs to be tailored to the symptoms of individuals. The basic philosophy behind treatment decisions is to reduce or eliminate physical activities that produce the new symptoms. This may of course require changing familiar routines at home and work. It may also necessitate using assistive devices such as canes, crutches, wheelchairs and scooters, or ventilators.[8] The key is working with a knowledgeable physician to preserve muscle function and reduce pain and fatigue while pursuing those activities important to the individual. Since the symptoms of post-polio syndrome can worsen over time, and since new symptoms can develop, devising effective treatment needs to be an evolving process involving both the polio survivor and his or her physician.

Coping with the symptoms of post-polio syndrome means dealing with both the physical changes in the body and with the psychological impact of a new disability. Polio survivors who made a good recovery in the forties and fifties, who finished their educations, had careers, married, and raised families often did not consider themselves to be disabled. Inconvenienced perhaps, but not disabled. When post-polio symptoms, or the recommended treatments, required individuals to give up meaningful and lucrative work, to abandon enjoyable leisure activities, or leave household chores undone, the psychological impact could be significant. Thus part of dealing with post-polio syndrome is finding ways to cope psychologically as well as physically.[9]

Just as a case of acute poliomyelitis involved the entire family, so too does the development of post-polio syndrome. Family members have to take on tasks that the polio survivor can no longer perform. They may also need to begin to help their spouse or parent with some of the activities of daily living such as getting dressed, taking a shower, getting up in the morning, and going to bed at night. Perhaps the house needs to be modified to accommodate a wheelchair or scooter. Perhaps an early retirement is necessary, leaving the spouse to provide the family's income. And since, as we noted above, there is often a psychological dimension when post-polio syndrome develops, family members may have to deal with anger, frustration, and depression as the polio survivor tries to adjust to the changes imposed by the new symptoms. Spouses, in particular, sometimes have difficulty accepting the changes brought by post-polio syndrome since they can affect earning potential, household responsibilities, and sexual intimacy. While many spouses and families adjust well to changed circumstances, others have found it difficult to accept the new limitations on the polio survivor and the new responsibilities they need to take up.

Many polio survivors thought they had put polio behind them when they walked or wheeled into the American mainstream in the fifties and sixties. Physical therapy and surgery were finished and they were encouraged to get on with their lives. They found effective ways to deal with the physical limitations left by polio. Most expected that their polio-related problems would remain relatively stable over their lifetimes. But polio was not something that one left behind. At the end of the twentieth century survivors discovered that they were not done living with polio. New lessons had to be learned—"use it and lose it" instead of "use it or lose it." They would have to renegotiate the worlds of home, family, and work.

Onset, Symptoms, and Diagnosis

Margo Vickery contracted polio in New Jersey in 1946 when she was five years old.

Ten years ago I was totally free. I could do anything that I wanted to do, anytime that I wanted to do. I knew about post-polio syndrome because my mother had sent me an article out of the newspaper. It was about a post-polio group. There was a doctor mentioned in there, whose name I don't remember. I was very busy working and I didn't have any effects yet. I just kind of let it go.

It was almost overnight that I had post-polio syndrome. It began with an episode, in which I experienced a severe emotional trauma, and the next day I couldn't even pick up a book. I was so weak, and I was in a lot of pain. I went to my doctor, and he prescribed Percodan for the pain. He really didn't try to discover what the matter was. I was running a company and going to graduate school at the same time. For the next five years, I took Percodan round the clock every six hours. I thought, "This isn't getting me anywhere." It allowed me to get through graduate school, but once that was over, I said, "Enough of this," and I changed doctors.

The next doctor that I went to was very nice. Nobody knew anything about post-polio. By this time, I was bringing it up, and I said, "Could this be something?" He said, "No. This isn't post-polio. You have some arthritis. We'll treat you for arthritis." I do have arthritis. I still wasn't satisfied. I was in a lot of pain, getting weaker. It's a very strange feeling. You don't know what's happening to you, and when you try to go to someone who's supposed to know about these things, you're treated as if you're crazy. I went through a series of doctors.

During this time, my right arm stopped functioning totally after some extremely severe pain. I was away, and I went to a doctor in California. He said, "Oh, don't worry about it. We'll just give you something for the pain." I didn't take care of it; the pain was gone, but I couldn't move my arm. When I came back home, the doctor wouldn't even let me out of his office before he got an appointment with a neurosurgeon. I had some tests done, and the neurosurgeon wanted to do surgery on my spine. I said, "Can you fix it?" He said, "I'm really not sure." I said, "Thank you very much."

I was being told that this was arthritis. I know a lot of people with arthritis, and they don't have the problems that I have. It didn't make sense.

When I first had polio I felt extremely fortunate because once I was over the disease, I didn't really "live" with polio. It really wasn't a part of my life. The only thing I remember is gratitude. During the time that I was growing up, you would see more people than you do now with withered limbs or braces, and each time I would see someone, I would feel very grateful.

When I was finally diagnosed with post-polio syndrome, I was thinking, "Hallelujah. I have an answer." One day, I thought to myself, "I'm going to search on the web and put in 'post-polio syndrome.' I probably won't get any hits." There were 1,200 hits. I almost fell off the chair.

I started reading web pages and found people writing the same kinds of things that I had experienced. I found people whose doctors didn't know anything about it, and even if no one came out and said you're crazy, they looked at you kind of askance. I sat there in front of the computer and just cried.

Through that research, I found Dr. Julie Silver; she's the one that diagnosed me with post-polio syndrome after doing tests and ruling out everything else. I wrote out my history and gave it to her because a lot of times you don't remember. She sat there and carefully read the whole thing, which was amazing to me, coming from doctors that you're maybe allowed fifteen minutes if you're lucky. There was this caring feeling. When she did tell me that's what it was, certainly it's not something I wanted, but now I had an answer.

Edward O'Connor contracted polio in Bronx, NY, in 1955 when he was ten years old.

About three years or four years ago I began noticing I don't sleep good. My back hurts, and my right leg hurts, and I used to be very strong. I used to workout a lot. I'm not half as strong as I used to be. I could really lift and do whatever I wanted. It just shuts me down.

Ted Kellogg contracted polio in Westfield, MA, in 1943 when he was five and a half years old.

When the news filtered out about post-polio, I basically wrote it off because I was feeling good. I never felt better in my life than after I passed forty years old. Within a couple of years, I started noticing increased weakness. I started reading about post-polio. There was a rehabilitation doctor at the Bay State Medical Center in Springfield, Massachusetts who sent out flyers to polio folks and had a seminar on a Sunday afternoon. After the seminar, I made an appointment with him. He told me enough about it for me to know that it's happening to me.

I'm naturally right-handed, and polio did a weird thing to me. My right arm has always been weaker than my left arm, but my right hand was always stronger than my left hand, and so that enabled me to stay right-handed. Since the mid-eighties, my right arm and hand are just about worthless. If there's something on a table, I have to throw my arm at it and hope I latch onto it, or else go further into the room, turn around, come back and get it with my left hand. As unbelievable as this may sound, I notice an increased weakness in my right leg, which nobody sees me move anyway because I am paralyzed in my legs and use a wheelchair. There is just a little bit of movement in my right leg compared to my left leg, but now my right leg feels tired all the time.

Bill Schweid, M.D., contracted polio in Okinawa, Japan, in 1947 when he was twenty-five years old.

The physicians, they're totally stupid about post-polio in my opinion. My orthopedist knows about it. When he was in training, his teachers told him about polio, but he didn't see it. He's in his early fifties. He didn't see any polio, but he said, "I now see post-polio problems." Many doctors don't know what post-polio syndrome is. They think they've learned everything and know everything anyway, so why bother. That's the attitude of many physicians. Some think people are neurotic who have post-polio symptoms.

Justine Guckin contracted polio in Newington, CT, in 1969 when she was two years old.

About ten years ago, my mother came across an Ann Landers column, which mentioned post-polio syndrome. They had a phone number to call. I called them because I was starting to get tired a lot more and noticeably more pain. It's not like one day you can walk, and one day you can't; it's a slow progression. It feels like you're getting old a lot faster than everybody else around you, and it's scary because you don't know what the next step is going to be. It's like, "My legs are going. Are my arms going to go, too? Am I going to not be able to do this next year, if I'm doing it this year? Will I be able to go Christmas shopping this year? Wow, if I don't have my wheelchair and I don't have my van, how the heck am I going to get around? Where can we go for dinner that doesn't have any stairs?" I think it's just the fear of the unknown.

Because it is a slow progression, I didn't know what was happening. Why does my good leg hurt all of a sudden? Why am I in so much pain? Why am I so tired? I thought it was going to get bad faster. It did get bad fast, but I thought that it was going to be worse than it actually is. It's all in who you work with, though. My polio support group is a huge part of my life.

EFFECT ON THE FAMILY

Richard Rosenwald, M.D., contracted polio in Framingham, MA, in 1956 when he was thirty-two years old.

I have had a hard time with post-polio syndrome. I fell in 1988. I slipped and fractured my hip. I had, in the past, fractured my kneecap twice on the bad leg. The first time, I was rushing to a meeting downtown in the State Building, and my feet went out from under me, and I came down on my right knee. At the meeting my knee swelled up, and I went off to the emergency room, had X-rays and a cast put on. Then I fractured it again. I just tripped over a little step that I didn't see in a store and went down on the knee, and it fractured again. I've been using a respirator since 1996. I'm in a wheelchair now. I have serious shortness of breath. I have new weakness, have trouble standing up from chairs and bed.

I'm in a nursing home now. My wife, whose polio was worse than mine, and I got to the point that we just couldn't manage the house anymore. For the first few years after we had polio I would take care of her on Sunday and Saturday afternoon. We just used to get teenagers to come in Sunday morning. We had a lady from Jamaica, Millie, for ten years. We had her daughter, Ann, for four years. She was wonderful, took great care of Marsha. When she left, the help situation just fell apart. We started having all kinds of trouble, and Marsha got very depressed, both over losing Ann and over feeling she wasn't going to be taken care of. I was able to do less to help out. That frightened her, too. We were very worried that something would happen to me and she'd be left alone.

Marsha had given up. She couldn't cope anymore. We chose to go into a nursing home together. Marsha had a terrible time. She was very controlling and she was used to having her own personal aide. It's not like that in the nursing home. They have one aide per ten people. You've got to share. They don't come right away. Marsha was always panicky.

Marsha was starting to deteriorate a little bit in terms of post-polio. Her breathing was getting a little worse. The depression was debilitating, and it just didn't respond to medication. She couldn't adjust to the nursing home.

In the nursing home, our daughter, Betsy, planned a fiftieth wedding anniversary party for us. For two weeks prior to the party, Marsha talked about what she would wear. On the day of the party, I got one of the aides to attend to Marsha. The party was great. Marsha was happy, like the old Marsha. She had a great time. That night we both went to bed, and about quarter of twelve the lights went out, and the generator failed, and Marsha didn't make it.

She seemed okay at first. The nurses were calling 911, calling the administrator to find out what to do. I was with Marsha, trying to reassure her it would be all right. She asked me for the blower, and I just shook my head. A few minutes later, she said, "Help! Help! I can't breathe!" and just went out and went limp. I yelled to the nurses, "Help! Help! Call 911!" One of them came right down and realized she wasn't breathing. Another one came in, and they started CPR. A few minutes later the paramedics came. They didn't seem to be able to do anything.

She went to the hospital. They got her breathing and her heart going again, but her blood pressure just wouldn't come up. The doctors told me that there wasn't anything they could do to save her. I keep asking myself, was there anything I could have or should have done? It's not easy. I still wake up from time to time and think she's still beside me.

George Durr contracted polio in Peekskill, NY, in 1931 when he was eighteen months old.

I can't drive anymore. I used to love that I could drive the car. I drove a Model T car, which had three pedals in it. It had a brake, a clutch and a reverse, which I did with one foot. People couldn't figure out how I could manage. Being dependent on my wife to take me somewhere is my biggest thing right now. The sickness itself never bothered me to any extent. I'm grateful for every day that I'm doing something, because I never expected that things would turn this good for me.

We play the lottery, and I said to my wife, "Even if we won the lottery, what would we do differently? There's nothing I would want to do differently."

William Zanke contracted polio in Wheeling, WV, in 1949 or 1950 when he was four years old.

I think it has some effect on my wife. I think she worries about me. I'm not sure it has much of an impact on my kids. My two children, sixteen and eighteen, still see me as indestructible and will go on forever. My son understands we can't wrestle anymore, and part of that's more about him getting big than me getting old. My kids are starting to see that I'm wearing out some, but I don't think they really internalize that much.

Mike Pierce contracted polio in Southington, CT, in 1949 when he was five and a half years old.

I was a civil engineer, so I did the civil works for the oil companies, building roads, bridges, pipelines, mechanical features, did a few airfields, houses. I worked for the state of Connecticut as the bridge engineer, and was responsible for one-quarter of the state. My career ended when I had to go out on disability because the state could not find any position for me. Post-polio syndrome cut my career short by twelve to fourteen years. When I went out on disability my wife told me, "You know, I could understand if you had cancer, but you look fine to me. Why retire?" I just tried to explain to her that I couldn't work anymore. I couldn't walk beams. I'd be falling down embankments. I know I got a pretty good life insurance policy, but I don't want the kids to collect it that way. I was just hit on all ends at one time, going through being diagnosed as post-polio, trying to find out what was wrong with me, the job, the home life. Everything fell to pieces. I was 56 years old.

My wife totally freaked out. I think she had a nervous breakdown. She lost confidence in me as a husband, as a provider, but with the disability and the retirement coming in, it was a fairly sizable income. I'd still be able to contribute; she was working also. We had a nice house and lots of acreage, a couple of big dogs and two kids that were growing up. I was still quite active at the time.

At the time of my retirement, my son was playing tennis. I knew a lot of the coaches, and they knew what I was going through. The coaches didn't tell me they were going to do this, but one day they announced in school that "There is something wrong with Mr. Pierce, and he's got polio. We're going to dedicate the tennis season to Mike's dad, Mr. Pierce." This announcement totally freaked out my daughter. Everyone was coming up and sobbing, and she came back to me screaming and saying, "I've lost everything. I've lost my friends and you've got this thing."

She was against me, the wife was against me, and my son was torn between the two sides. Eventually I lost everything. The wife, the daughter, the son, they were turned against me, the dogs, the house, everything that I'd worked for. If I could have just worked until I was sixty-seven, max sixty-nine I was going to retire. I'd have enough left over for the wife and us to live comfortably. She was twelve years younger than I was, and all she could see was that she had to work another twenty years to support a family. She didn't realize that I was still supporting our family with my disability income.

I hope to reconcile with my kids. I don't think I'll ever be able to reconcile with the wife. She was too set on getting out from everything and everybody. She still had another twenty years to work, and she didn't want to go around supporting me. It also didn't help that one of her best friends is married to a paraplegic, a guy with multiple sclerosis, and he's completely wheelchair-bound. The stories that they used to tell about him behind his back. My wife just didn't want to wind up like that, caring for a guy that would mess his pants. Once she heard that I could progress into a wheelchair, she wanted nothing of it.

I would have really hurt myself bad if I didn't stop working. I thought it was time to look after myself, see if I could get myself a few extra years and not go into a wheelchair or be totally incapacitated. I'm striving for that now. Probably I will stay out of a wheelchair, and I will live to ninety-seven or more. I've set the goal and I'll make it. Even if I've got to crawl, I'll make it.

The worst thing about post-polio syndrome is losing what you invested, twenty-one years of your life and seeing your kids grow up and losing that. I just lost my whole world. But, I'm going to climb back up that ladder. I'm not going to give up.

Ted Kellogg contracted polio in Westfield, MA, in 1943 when he was five and a half years old.

My wife and I are beginning to face the normal problems of aging. She's a small woman. She weighs 114 pounds. She's always been a dynamo that can't sit still, but she's having to help me do little insignificant things like pick up something off the floor. That's how post-polio can affect you. I can't easily pick things up off the floor anymore because my right arm isn't strong enough to hold me in the wheelchair as I lean over to pick it up with my left.

CHANGES IN QUALITY OF LIFE

Jody Leigh Griffin contracted polio in Anchorage, AK, in 1954 when she was three years old.

I'm a master gardener. Projects that I had taken on in the past, I wasn't willing to take on because it took a lot out of me. This year I'm really avoiding doing things that I wouldn't have thought even twice about before. My husband loves gardening. He has no problem doing the things that save energy for me so that I can continue doing what I want to do. My son helps, too. He's come out and taken on projects because my husband's been sick. I have to balance things that need to be done and have to be done.

I started learning about post-polio and learned that pushing wasn't going to accomplish anything. Once I had that information, I had to shift the way I thought about things. I always thought, if you can imagine it, you can make it happen. If it makes demands on my body, then I have to start thinking, "Is this just about my mind and a desire, or does this mean that I have to put a demand on my body?"

I used to horseback ride and ride snowmobiles and motorcycles and hike in the White Mountains. Instead of pushing to accomplish a project today, I'd put it off and do it over the course of three or four days or maybe I just wouldn't do it at all. I had to change the way I thought and looked at life.

I regret that there are things that I will never do in this lifetime, but I know that having polio has tempered me, enlightened me, made me more sensitive and aware of other people. Without it I definitely might have been the self-centered gratification-oriented person that's inside there. I like who I became, rather than who I imagine I might have been.

My family, my parents, my grandparents, and everybody that was involved in my life, without them, it definitely would have been a different experience. I hate to use the word lucky, but on a spiritual level, there's definitely somebody watching and that's guided me through the dark places.

Justine Guckin contracted polio in Newington, CT, in 1969 when she was two years old.

When I was younger, and my kids were little, having polio was no big deal. I had polio; I wore a brace. Now it's different. I lost touch with a couple of friends because their view of my polio is, "Well, why are you giving up, and why are you going in a wheelchair? You used to be such a fighter. You used to do roller-skating and you used to downhill ski." It's so hard to explain things to some people. Sometimes people just don't want to listen. Can't you just accept that I'm going to be going from walking with just a brace to walking with a different brace with crutches or even in a wheelchair all the time? It's still me, it's still my heart, it's still my soul, it's still my body. I just kind of grab tighter to the friends that I still do have. My fiancé, Barron, is awesome. He's been a huge support. I've never had anybody besides my mother care and want to do so much for me. Even yell at me but not in a bad way, "Sit down and let me get that for you," and, "Why did you just do that?" The other night I moved the fan from the kitchen to the living room. Little, stupid plastic, very lightweight, but it was the point of getting up, going in the other room, getting it, and bringing it in the living room. Barron just looked at me and said, "Why didn't you just ask me to do that?"

Stephen Burwick contracted polio in Worcester, MA, in 1954 when he was twelve years old.

The worst thing about polio is that it hasn't gone away. It comes back to haunt me in my everyday life more and more, from falling and having broken my femur to having to wear a brace. I'm on about my fourth or fifth brace now. Every day I'm waiting to find out what's going on with my back and whether I need surgery. Every time I get more medical issues, I suspect that they're all interrelated to having polio. I think being overweight is related to having polio, just not getting enough exercise. I still have pain and discomfort.

If somebody had to have it, then it might as well have been me. It was the single most important experience in my life. Every time I feel sorry for myself, I always figure somebody's worse off. There were people that didn't make it. There were people in iron lungs.

Polio's a bitch. It strikes you down physically, but not mentally. You know what you can do, or what you want to do, and you just can't do it. It would be almost better if you didn't know how bad off you were.

COPING

William Zanke contracted polio in Wheeling, WV, in 1949 or 1950 when he was four years old.

I am not handling having post-polio syndrome very well. My primary coping mechanism for most of my life about polio was to ignore it. From the time in high school, if I would see a film of me playing football, the first reaction that I got was "Who the fuck is that?" I didn't see myself limping. I know it sounds contradictory. I never consciously thought much about having polio. It was only in a dating situation that I would think about the limp, and then not really very consciously. It was only later in life that I could see it. The physical pain that was involved I mostly dealt with by ignoring it.

Denial gets a bad rap because there's a lot of nice things that can happen to you around denial. Denial used to be an effective tool. After forty years of going without one, I wear a brace again. I'm now using a cane, which has an effect on the way people treat you. The limp has gotten worse. The day I started using a cane, the same guys who were knocking me over to try to beat me out of a door, now holding the door for me.

I'm having a lot of pain in different areas related to the polio, and I have a non-stable situation, which means that the physical condition that I have today is likely to get worse, not better, and there's nothing I can do to change that. The future may be mildly worse, or it may be a lot worse. I'm somebody who likes to feel like I have some power to impact things.

I fought getting that handicapped tag for parking for years because I didn't see myself as handicapped, and I didn't think it was an appropriate term to describe what my situation was. I realized that's not factually accurate, but it is how I felt about it.

Margo Vickery contracted polio in New Jersey in 1946 when she was five years old.

I'm not angry about having had polio. I don't know whether I'm angry about post-polio. "Angry" isn't the word. Disappointed, depressed, feeling like I'm not contributing anything. That's from post-polio syndrome, not from the polio.

The effects of polio can be so long-range. It isn't just during the time that you have the active disease. Through research and through education, the medical community, I'm sure, can come up with things that can make life better for people with post-polio syndrome. I emphasize that so much more because that's what's affected my life much more than the polio did.

Bill Schweid, M.D., contracted polio in Okinawa, Japan, in 1947 when he was twenty-five years old.

I am grateful and feel quite humbled having developed polio at age twenty-five because it has provided me with a lot of insight as a physician to understand how other people feel. I never wanted to be a surgeon because my skill is in communicating. People have often said to me, "I tell you things I've never told anybody else. I feel comfortable talking to you." When I interview patients my first comment to them is, "I am not God. I do make errors, but I do listen to people and I do not discourage you from talking, and if I talk too much that's bad, I learn more by listening." There are many physicians who are quite brilliant and they know everything in the literature and the latest modes of treatment, but they don't ask the patient, "Did you understand me?" or, "What did you hear?" I've been humbled having to deal with polio and post-polio syndrome. I feel I've been a better person and a better physician and healer having had this type of experience.

Edward O'Connor contracted polio in Bronx, NY, in 1955 when he was ten years old.

The worst thing about having post-polio syndrome is that my physical problems are slowing me down. There was really no real starting point that I could really say, "Wow, my life's in turmoil on account of this." I have a very aggressive personality. In the past, every job that I wanted, I went and I got. If I had to torture people, aggravate people, annoy people, call them up, lie on my eye test, whatever it took, the ones that I wanted, I got. Maybe my having had polio had something to do with it. Maybe that made me more aggressive.

Ruth Esau contracted polio in Cass City, MI, in 1919 when she was two years old.

I left teaching unhappily. I had a very cruel principal. I left suddenly in 1972. That was the beginning of post-polio. I shouldn't have gone back that year. I stayed only thirteen days. Instead of talking to me, she removed all my perks, all the things that were making it easy for me. During the summer I wrote to her and said I didn't ever want to be treated like that again. When I went back in the fall, she just didn't speak to me. She took away the bathroom privileges, and she took my aide away from me. I should have filed a grievance, but I didn't. I just knew I couldn't work with her anymore.

Judy Lappin contracted polio in Swampscott, MA, in 1953 when she was five years old.

Having post-polio syndrome has made me mad. I felt like my whole life I had polio, and I conquered it. I thought I was going to be fine the rest of my life. It feels a little bit like a double whammy. I've used some denial. That's not going to happen to me for a while and wanting to believe that because I was so functional that it wasn't going to happen to me; it was going to happen to the people who were in worse shape. It's been very difficult because nobody has real clear answers about how much is enough and how much is too much. Ignored it in terms of not wanting to limit my activity. It's kind of been a process. I probably should have cut back on my exercise sooner.

My mother will often say to me things like do you think you're exercising too much, which leads me to believe that she's read about it, but would never bring it up.

Dorothy Arnold contracted polio in Massachusetts in 1947 when she was twenty-three years old.

About ten years or so ago, I would be running up to the net playing tennis, and I'd find that I was sort of out of breath. I asked my doctor, "What's the story? I'm running up to the net and I'm not as fast as I used to be." He said, "Dorothy, come on." If I'm eighty now, it was when I was about seventy. I had all those years in between with not a whisper of polio.

Fatigue is the biggest thing. I lie down at ten-thirty, sometimes for ten or twenty minutes, and then I get up and have lunch at twelve o'clock with my husband. I always have a nap in the afternoon, which to me is a waste of time, but totally necessary. I come back to my art studio for an hour or so, and then go home and have an early dinner with my husband.

I'm not angry about having had polio, but I have anger about the fact that I fought it once, and now why the hell does it have to come back and tap me on the shoulder?

Noreen Abbot contracted polio in California in 1953 when she was three years old.

My mother was very upset. All she could think about was what did she do to make me so ill. She doesn't like to talk about it. To her polio's something bad, something awful. It's something that should not be spoken about. My mother's from China, and my father died a few months before I had polio. I was the only child, and it was just a very hard time for her.

She does know that the polio weakened me, but she does not understand the post-polio syndrome. I'm not going to even try to explain it to her because my Chinese is not that good, and she doesn't really want to hear about it. She would say, "Oh, we all get weak as we get old." That may be true for some people, but they can always exercise and try to regenerate certain muscles and muscle tone. But not with polio.

For my mother post-polio syndrome is difficult. Even to see me in the wheelchair today, it's difficult. She cannot understand how my husband can accept it. She feels I should be very good to him because I am handicapped, and if I do anything wrong, he will run off with an able-bodied woman. That relates back to her own culture. In the Chinese culture a man is free to do whatever he wants. Especially if you are a crippled wife, he has every right to leave you, and chances are he could leave you because of the way you are.

Kathleen Givant contracted polio in California in 1946 when she was eight years old.

I worry about not overextending myself because I do have some post-polio now. It's affecting me a lot in that, for one thing, I don't go shopping anymore. I view myself as still being fairly young in some respects, but my body feels a lot older than my mind feels. When I get up in the morning, I try to do everything I can in the first half of the day because the second half of the day I get very tired.

Some of my friends who are my age will take trips to Europe. I don't think I have the stamina to do it. I don't want to be a burden on anybody. I don't want people to have to wait for me. I choose not to do that kind of thing. Post-polio syndrome certainly has changed my leisure, but I don't consider it a burden because I choose to do other things.

I watched my father deteriorate. He had a ton of post-polio.

8

POLIO TODAY AND ITS EFFECT ON ADVANCES IN MEDICINE

Most American polio survivors are now in their fifties, or older, and their numbers are being reduced every year. Children today have no memory of those fear-ridden years, and in most cases no memory of receiving the vaccine that protects them from the disease. Recent books and documentary films have brought to the fore the memories of polio survivors and of the doctors, nurses, and physical therapists who cared for them.[1] The polio epidemics, however, significantly influenced the development of American medicine. The thousands of patients needing care and rehabilitation helped create the profession of physical therapy. The need to provide respiratory assistance to some polio survivors led first to the development of the iron lung and later to smaller and more portable means of artificial ventilation. This large cohort also spurred improvements in bracing, in orthopedic surgery, and in the development of assistive technologies. Techniques of viral culture pioneered by John Enders, Thomas Weller, and Frederick Robbins proved to be of value in growing viruses other than the poliovirus.[2] The magnitude of the polio epidemics, the large number of patients needing care and rehabilitation, and the funds provided by the National Foundation for Infantile Paralysis (NFIP) all provided an opportunity to innovate with important consequences for the advancement of medicine.

Although wild poliovirus has been gone from the western hemisphere for more than two decades, and is now restricted to a handful of countries in Africa and Asia, polio has not been completely eliminated from the concerns of physicians and scientists. The World Health Organization (WHO), supported by the fund-raising efforts of Rotary International and the Gates Foundation, remains committed to the effort to eradicate polio in the next several years. Even if their effort succeeds, new problems will appear. Should research stocks of the poliovirus be maintained? How long should immunization against polio be continued? Does the poliovirus have the potential to be used as a weapon of bioterrorism?

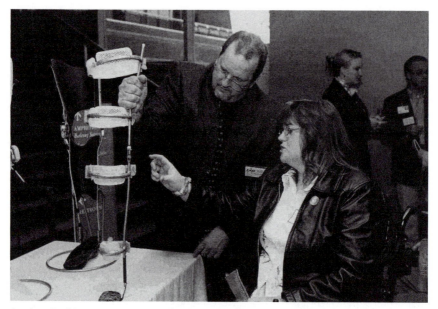

Justine Guckin comments on a leg brace displayed at a Polio Survivors Reunion in Boston in 2005. The event marked the 50th anniversary of the polio vaccine. Guckin contracted polio in 1969, when she was 2 years old. Photo courtesy of Justine Guckin.

The polio epidemics, along with the casualties of World War I, played important roles in the development of physical therapy as a specialized field and profession. In 1914 Dr. Robert Lovett, an orthopedic surgeon in Boston, began to train physiotherapists to work with polio patients. Many of these young women had some prior preparation in physical education, and Lovett provided additional instruction in "muscle training, corrective exercise, and massage," and in the use of muscle charts to measure and record muscle strength.[3] A short while later, the U.S. Army employed physical therapists in the rehabilitation of soldiers wounded in World War I. Mary McMillan, an English trained therapist, wrote the first book by a physical therapist published in the United States, *Massage and Therapeutic Exercise* (1921).[4] Managing the rehabilitation of hundreds of thousands of polio survivors, even more than the battle casualties, "created a unique void in the medical arena—a void that was filled by the rapid expansion of the profession of physical therapy."[5] Thus the dual tragedies of epidemic polio and war gave rise to physical therapy.

Franklin Roosevelt's development of a polio rehabilitation facility at Warm Springs, Georgia, in the late 1920s also contributed to the development of rehabilitation medicine. Several of the first generation of physical therapists, including Alice Lou Plastridge, worked at Warm Springs and transformed it from a resort into a leading rehabilitation facility. As its reputation grew, physical therapists from across the nation came to Georgia for training, the brace shop became known for its innovations, and new techniques in hydrotherapy were developed.[6]

The late twenties also saw the development of one of the most familiar, and feared, devices associated with the polio epidemics, the iron lung. Philip Drinker, an engineer at Harvard, built his first crude prototype in 1928. Drinker first tried the machine on cats, and later on himself and his colleagues. The first actual patient to use an iron lung was an eight-year-old girl paralyzed by polio. The iron lung sustained the girl for five days before she died of an unrelated infection. Drinker soon assigned the patent to the Warren E. Collins Company of Boston and the iron lung went into production. As David Rothman points out, the machine went from prototype to production and clinical use with almost no testing for safety or efficacy. Most of the early uses of the iron lung were in emergency situations where the patient would have died without the machine. Over time, with more machines, more patients, and more experience, physicians became more comfortable using them. However, serious ethical concerns marked the first decade of the iron lung. Would patients ever be able to be taken out of the machine and be able to breathe on their own? Was it ethical to risk condemning a patient to a lifetime in an iron lung? In addition, in the years before the development of antibiotics, a large number of patients in iron lungs succumbed to other infections.[7]

The establishment of the NFIP in 1938 helped to disseminate this new technology nationally and to train doctors to use iron lungs appropriately and successfully. The NFIP in the early forties purchased iron lungs and distributed them across the nation. By the late forties the NFIP had in place a quasi-military operation capable of quickly moving iron lungs across the country to any community experiencing a polio epidemic. Their enthusiastic promotion of the new technology, and their ability to deliver machines, increased demand for iron lungs.[8] In 1950 the NFIP counted 583 patients in 135 hospitals dependent on iron lungs for more than a month. Then, in order "to provide more expert care and to reduce costs, the NFIP established fifteen regional respirator centers." These centers conducted research in respiratory therapy, trained medical personnel to use the machines properly, and treated the most serious cases. Over time, many of these patients were able to go home even with their iron lungs, others were totally freed from dependence on respirators, or were able to use smaller, more portable respirators. Individuals have lived for years dependent on iron lungs for at least part of the day, but others died within a few years of leaving the respirator centers.[9] Even today, a few polio survivors still depend on the iron lung.[10]

The shortcomings of the iron lungs spurred the development of other means of artificial respiration. The late forties saw the development of the rocking bed that rocked like a teeter-totter with the patient lying on the mattress. When the head swung up, the internal organs moved downward pulling the diaphragm with them and pulling air into the lungs. When the feet swung up, the process was reversed. The rocking bed helped wean patients from iron lungs. Patients felt freer on the rocking bed and nurses found caring for the patients much easier.[11] Chest respirators were also developed in the late forties and early fifties. With these smaller, more portable respirators, patients could lie on a regular bed and even sit up or use a wheelchair. Some patients even figured out how to have sexual intercourse while using a chest respirator. Rocking beds and chest respirators were less effective than iron lungs, but they were a means of getting out of the iron lung and ultimately out of the hospital.[12]

The shortcomings of these negative pressure devices and the shortage of iron lungs spurred the development of positive pressure respirators. One of the first times that physicians used positive pressure respiration on a large scale was the 1952 polio epidemic in Copenhagen, Denmark. Soon new machines were developed and put into production. Positive pressure respirators work by forcing air into the lungs through the nose, mouth, or a tracheostomy. These machines were generally smaller than the negative pressure machines and were more efficient than rocking beds or cuirass respirators. They could be used by individuals wearing normal clothing, sitting up, or using a wheelchair, and they allowed the patients greater mobility. According to David Rothman, the development of positive pressure ventilation made it possible for surgeons to maintain "patients' respiratory functioning during and immediately after surgery." This opened the way for many innovative heart and lung surgeries. It also led to the development of intensive care units where many, if not all, of the patients were on respirators.[13]

The polio epidemic and its survivors also spurred the development of other devices to compensate for paralyzed muscles. These included lightweight plastic braces to replace the heavy steel and leather braces of the epidemic years. They also fostered the development of improved wheelchairs, including lightweight chairs, powered chairs, and scooters. The needs of polio survivors encouraged the development of "environmental controls" such as microswitches, computers, and other devices to manipulate their environment and to compensate for a lack of muscle strength.[14] The many casualties of World War II, Korea, and Vietnam, as well as the growing number of automobile accident survivors, also provided incentives to improvise and a market for assistive devices. Still, polio survivors were important in the development of new and improved medical technology.

Funding from the NFIP also paid for advanced training for physical therapists, nurses, and other health professionals. For example, in 1955 Dr. Hart Van Riper, Medical Director of NFIP, estimated that the Foundation had supported the training of one third of the 6,000 physical therapists then working in the United States. In the 1940s and 1950s the NFIP also provided funds to improve the training of nurses, especially in orthopedic and public health nursing. The NFIP also allotted funds to train African American physicians, nurses, and physical therapists. The organization provided over one million dollars to establish and maintain the Infantile Paralysis Center at Tuskegee Institute to train black health professionals to care for polio patients. Many of "these benefits were transferred to persons with other crippling diseases" after the Salk and Sabin vaccines ended the polio epidemics.[15]

Even the famous 1954 Polio Vaccine Trial of the Salk vaccine had an impact on subsequent field trials of experimental vaccines. Donald Burke, a professor of public health at Johns Hopkins, has recently identified several lessons learned from the 1954 Salk trial. These lessons include the realization that large, even very large, trials are possible, but that they require "committed, effective leadership" to succeed. Burke believes Basil O'Connor's leadership and commitment brought all the pieces together successfully. The ability of the NFIP to organize and fund the trial made it clear that nongovernmental organizations could succeed at such an undertaking. But even a successful trial "is just a beginning." As Burke notes, fifty years after the trial was successfully concluded, polio eradication remains an elusive goal.[16]

In early 2005, wild poliovirus still had not been eradicated, and because of political and religious problems in Nigeria, 2004 saw an actual increase of polio cases in Africa. Whereas 2003 had only 447 cases of polio in Africa, there were 1,037 in 2004. In 2003 there were only three African countries that had not stopped the transmission of polio, Egypt, Niger, and Nigeria, but because polio immunization was halted for most of a year in northern Nigeria, five nearby countries reported polio cases in 2004.[17] These recent problems illustrate the challenges facing the WHO and its allies in their efforts to eradicate polio from its last reservoirs in Africa and Asia.[18] Donald Henderson, who led the successful effort to eradicate smallpox, suggests that polio vaccination will need to continue in most countries into the foreseeable future because polio is proving more difficult to eradicate than smallpox.[19]

While some concerns have been raised about the potential of the poliovirus to become a weapon of bioterrorism, the WHO argues that the poliovirus is a "poor" choice "for use in biological warfare or acts of bioterrorism, because the vast majority of poliovirus infections (>99%) would not result in paralytic manifestations, even in a susceptible population." However, they also note that the "release of poliovirus into a highly susceptible population could greatly enhance public anxiety"[20] Thus, in spite of the best efforts of medical science and the WHO, polio is likely to remain a potential threat even in areas declared free of the disease, and immunization will need to continue worldwide for some time to come.

Although the threat of polio has receded for most Americans and in most countries of the world, the impact of polio and the twentieth-century epidemics continues. Polio was a hard teacher, but the lessons learned in the more than one hundred years of epidemic polio have improved the lives of polio survivors and others with similar impairments, spurred the creation of new assistive devices, and brought the poliovirus to the brink of extinction.

John Patrick Whelan, M.D., Ph.D., treated Jonas Salk in the last weeks of Salk's life.

My birthday is April 12th, 1960. I had an awareness through my growing-up years about the significance of the date of my own birth. Beyond the start of the Civil War; the other great significance of the date was that Franklin

[D.] Roosevelt had died on that day, and that in 1955 the results of the polio vaccine trials were released. Two of the three momentous occasions associated with April 12th had been polio-related.

As a child, one of the most significant experiences I had was being at a children's camp and being exposed there to another child who contracted polio, and having to get an immunoglobulin shot in my gluteal area afterwards. It made quite an impression on me. I had a significant awareness of polio, maybe more than most children of my era who were vaccinated for polio and didn't worry about it.

I did my graduate studies in immunology and went through an M.D./Ph.D. program at Baylor College of Medicine in Houston. I was the head teaching fellow for six years for the immunology course and I had an opportunity to develop a deeper understanding of the practical elements of immunity and how we acquire immunity. I had a lot of opportunity to think about vaccination, how vaccines work, and what it would take to develop an HIV vaccine. In that context I became well acquainted with Dr. [Jonas] Salk's work and also had a great admiration for him personally because of his stands on social issues.

The circumstances in which I did meet him were under some duress for him. Our acquaintance was relatively brief, but I was probably one of the last people to have substantial conversations with him before he died. I was a second-year medicine resident at Scripps and I was working one Saturday in June 1995 in the hospital. I remember thinking as I drove past the Salk Institute, "I really have to make a point of going over and just introducing myself to Dr. Salk one of these days." It's funny that I had that specific thought that morning.

It was the graduation day for our residency program. I was supposed to be off duty at three in the afternoon to attend a fancy graduation event down on the Coronado Island. Just as we were finishing up for the day, one of the cardiology fellows said that he had just gotten paged to our Urgent Care Center, that Dr. Salk had come in and wasn't feeling well and did I want to go with him. The cardiology fellow and I walked into the room where Dr. Salk was lying on a gurney. He just looked very fatigued. He wasn't short of breath, but he looked uncomfortable and yet very dignified. The cardiology fellow was a little bit anxious as we walked into the room. He introduced me to Dr. Salk by my last name. He said, "This is Dr. Whelan." I remember thinking that's a little formal, considering I'm a resident and this is Jonas Salk.

Another patient came into the Urgent Care Center, who was in the midst of an acute myocardial infarction, so the cardiology fellow had to leave, and he entrusted the patient to me. I sat down and did a thorough history and physical exam. Dr. Salk related to me how he had had a cardiac catheterization a few months earlier and had done very well after that. He had not been feeling well for several days the preceding week. I remember him telling me that he had gone to a reception of some kind the week before and had a plate of sushi and a lot of salty Japanese food. We speculated together that he had just overloaded himself from a salt and fluid standpoint and that was why he was having a little more difficulty breathing. It struck me at the time that this was something more serious because he hadn't been able to sleep for the last few nights. He was clearly very anxious.

The studies that he had done that day were reassuring. He had a normal EKG. He had cardiac enzymes that were normal. It appeared that he didn't have any new damage to his heart. We decided to admit him to the intensive care unit and treat him with medications to help get rid of some fluid and see if we could help his breathing.

At six the next morning I rounded on him; he was sitting up in bed. He was reading the paper, and he felt dramatically better. We hoped that somehow this was just a transient crisis. I probably spent about three and a half hours talking with Jonas Salk. I've often thought about the content of that conversation, which was the dream conversation for a young immunologist, visiting with somebody who he had long wanted to meet. His health was at the center of the conversation, at least at first. I remember mentioning to him that there had been a quote in the newspaper the day before from [Speaker of the House] Newt Gingrich, who when asked at a press conference if the government ever did anything right, he said, "Well, they do some things right, like curing polio." Dr. Salk just laughed and said, "The government didn't have anything to do with it." He talked a little bit about the March of Dimes and how substantial their support had been for his work before and since. He made a comment that there's always ennui in science about taking the next big step. There's an incrementalism about science where people want to do the safe next experiment. There's always a feeling that more research is required, and wariness about taking the big steps to actually implementing something and bringing it to some public usefulness. He said that was clearly the case with the polio vaccine where everybody was convinced that this was not ready for primetime; we needed more study. He said, "I decided to heck with that. I'm not going to let children continue to be afflicted by polio in the way that they have been, tens of thousands every year, year after year, when we have the means potentially to make the vaccine. Let's go ahead and do it. And I did it. Everybody's always been shocked that I didn't patent the vaccine. But how can you patent something like water or air, which is something that everybody needs? I could not have stomached profiting myself from the vaccine since it was so clear that it was so necessary to the well-being of everybody."

That day we just had this wonderful opportunity to get acquainted, and I really did feel extraordinarily fortunate to have had the chance to meet him. I went home that evening and came back in the following Monday morning and visited with him again. When he was ready to go, I wrote all his prescriptions. He and I sat next to the pharmacy together while he waited for his prescriptions to be filled. Everything seemed like it was going well. He paged me that afternoon from home. He had a question about one of his medications. He wasn't feeling well later in the afternoon and he actually came back and checked himself into the hospital that evening. He had a cardiac catheterization on that Tuesday morning; I got to watch the procedure. He had an angioplasty performed. They got a very good result with opening up one particular area of his heart that had been deprived of sufficient circulation. I had a chance to visit with him later in the day when he came out of the ICU; he was sleepy and still under conscious sedation. I came back the following morning, and he was sitting up in bed with this big sandbag in his lap. He said, "You just won't believe the sensation that I had when they opened up that blood vessel. It was as if a tide of well-being washed over me. It was extraordinary. It was supernatural. There was just something about it, it wasn't just that I could breathe easier, it was all of a sudden my whole outlook on life was dramatically improved in an instant. Thank you so much." I said, "Gosh, I had nothing to do with it."

On that Friday, he experienced a cardiac arrest in the Urgent Care Center and was rushed to the ICU. I was in the ICU that Friday morning. I heard this ominous ringing announcement over the hospital public address system, "Code Blue, ICU," and they gave his bed number. Code Blue is a cardiopulmonary arrest, and anybody who's on service at the time has to drop what they're doing and run over to be of assistance. It's unusual for them to call a code in the ICU because there are critical-care people there already.

I dropped what I was doing, and I walked into the room. It was a crushing sight to see, Jonas lying there in the bed surrounded by people with a sense of urgency. It was clear that heroic measures were taken to try and save him, but in the end, they were never able to overcome the electrolyte abnormalities, which had caused his cardiac arrest. He died that morning. I don't mean to over dramatize what role I had in his life. I was able to relate to him at a level of what his work was while he was in the hospital those last few days. I know that he felt a sense of ministering to me, that I was somebody whose career was ahead of him and that he clearly felt that he had a role to inspire, and he did inspire.

Ted Kellogg contracted polio in Westfield, MA, in 1943 when he was five and a half years old.

If someone came up for a cure for my paralysis, I would pass because it would create for me more problems than it would solve. I would take the added strength. It would help me transfer, but I wouldn't go that walking route today. I'm too old for new things. I was relieved when I initially had polio when they finally took the braces away from me and stopped standing me up where I could barely move. I always had a thing about being stared at, being the subject of attention. If I were to start walking now, I would more than likely have a weird gait. People have stared at me my whole life. I handle this now much better than I used to. When I was young, I was belligerent. If somebody tried to just offered to hold a door for me, I'd snarl, "I can get it myself!"

Justine Guckin contracted polio in Newington, CT, in 1969 when she was two years old.

I appreciate life a lot more. I appreciate every little thing that God has to offer 100 percent. Other people have learned to do this by watching me, especially even my kids. There're some days that I sit on my little "pity pot." I can still jump, sing, dance. Polio is still around. I think that it's just as much an emotional disability as it is a physical one. The more support people get, the better off they are, especially if they have a good support group behind them, whether it be family, friends, the medical staff, doctors, nurses, secretaries. It's hard to live with polio.

Ray Taylor contracted polio in Cincinnati, OH, in 1925 when he was nine months old.

My early recollection is my mother rubbing my legs at night with cocoa butter. I have no idea what the cocoa butter was all about, but it was undoubtedly believed that by rubbing my legs they were improving the circulation. This was in the thirties. My family never mentioned polio, and I suppose that was the way people looked at any kind of crippling or abnormal behavior in those days. You just ignored it. That was my defense. I just used denial. I said to myself, "There's nothing wrong with me. There's no reason I can't play basketball or baseball or whatever." I tried and did succeed to some extent.

I actually got interested in Rotary when I was a little boy. My dad had died when I was not quite six years old, and we had moved from Cincinnati to Sheridan, Indiana. One of my mentors was the father of one of my best friends. He was a Rotarian, so when they would have father and son things, he would invite me to go along as his surrogate son. I grew up thinking that Rotarian men were great people because they had nice meals and looked after guys.

It wasn't until I had retired in 1982 and come to Pinehurst, North Carolina that I had the opportunity to join. My reason for doing it at that time was the good feeling I'd built up through the years about Rotary. They were one of the few organizations I knew anything about that was actually interested in working toward world peace.

I became a club president, and Rotary came up with the Polio Plus Program, which was a fundraising drive. Our involvement was to be raising the money necessary to buy the vaccine, and then the vaccine was to be dispensed by United Nations groups such as the WHO [World Health Organization] and UNICEF [United Nations Children's Fund], and the Centers for Disease Control [and Prevention].

I was chosen to be a fundraising chairman for our local area. In our little club, we had about forty members and we raised $44,000, which was considerably above our quota. Rotary had set a quota 120 million, and we raised 220 million.

We want to be able to empower individual Rotarians wherever they are. They don't have to have a whole club project. Someone in a Rotary Club someplace might be able to find a wheelchair for somebody, might be able to take them to the doctor, or we will be publishing health bulletins that many people who do not have access to medical doctors can come to the website and learn from that. In the western world polio hasn't been seen for three or four decades, so we're helping to educate the medical profession that there are problems that go with the initial onset.

The thing that has made Rotary successful in the less developed countries, particularly those that have had tribal wars and wars of various kinds, no one is afraid of Rotarians. Mothers are willing to bring their babies into town, knowing that nobody's going to hurt them. There have been instances in Africa where warring factions have stopped for a day or two, at an agreed-on time, so that we can vaccinate the babies. That's the advantage that Rotary has; we don't threaten anybody and we're not political or religious. We're just trying to help the children of the world and their families.

Peter Carnevale, a Rotarian in Providence, RI, is involved in the polio eradication effort.

I've been involved with polio since 1985 when Rotary started their campaign against polio—trying to eradicate it from the world. Several years ago I finished being district governor. The incoming governor, Dan Williams, asked me if I would chair the Polio Eradication Fund. Our goal was to try to eradicate polio by 2005, which was the hundredth anniversary of Rotary. I took over the chairmanship and tried to raise money. We raised over four hundred thousand dollars from approximately sixty-five Rotary clubs in my area. This is way beyond our goal.

It was Rotary International's goal to rid the world of polio, along with the World Health Organization and the Center for Disease Control, and also UNICEF. We were challenged by Dr. Sabin in 1985, who created the vaccine that could be taken orally, to rid the world of polio. He predicted that some eight million children would perish in the next twenty years. When Rotary accepted Dr. Sabin's challenge, there were more than 350,000 cases of polio reported in 125 countries. In 2002, there were only 480 cases reported in ten countries. We have had some setbacks. Some parts of Nigeria would not accept a vaccine coming from the western world. The governments in some of those communities put out the word that this was the western world's way of reducing the population, so we had to fight that.

We had hoped to do it by 2005, but it looks more like 2008 before we will achieve the goal. We're about 99 percent there. That 1 percent is the most difficult. We must continue to remain vigilant and support the goal. Polio will be the second disease worldwide that has been completely eradicated, the first one being smallpox. We feel very proud of that.

Bruce Aylward, M.D., MPH, is a physician who is the Coordinator of Global Polio Eradication Initiative at WHO.

One of the great problems has been getting the world to fully embrace and implement strategies. I remember someone saying, "Here's a resolution to eradicate polio, and we're going to tie your hands behind your back." The original resolutions and the initial work was not in the spirit of the way the eradication program had been run in the Americas. From the very outset, the program had big problems in terms of just endorsement to go beyond routine immunization into these massive campaigns that are necessary to interrupt transmission. There were real problems in terms of getting different areas of the world to start. I don't think people appreciated what was required, early in the program. It took some time to get them there. One region implemented, then another region implemented, and it had to have this proof of principle in multiple parts of the world before other areas got started.

More recently, there's been chronic insufficient financing of the program. It's been at too low a level within the agencies responsible for it, without answering to the senior levels necessary to get the political will behind it. The reason you need big political will is that a polio campaign means you immunize every kid under the age of five on one day. You do it again a month later. You do it again, if necessary, a month after that and at multiple times in multiple years. That has massive financial and other resource costs. To mobilize those kind of resources, you need the highest level of political support in the country to say, "We believe this is a priority," and make it a priority, and then turn on the mechanisms of state. You need the information ministries, the transport ministries, et cetera. You can only do that if polio is at a high level in the organizations responsible for it, and it has direct access to people like a Director General of WHO. It's been just a vision of a recent couple of Director Generals in WHO that have raised it up to that level.

The other big issue has been convincing a lot of skeptics that it's a good thing to do. The world of public health has been its own worst enemy. There's been ferocious debate that flares and dies about the appropriateness of moving to eradication and investing the kind of resources needed to do that.

William Foege, M.D., M.P.H., is currently a fellow of the Bill & Melinda Gates Foundation. He's also the founder of the Task Force for Child Survival and Development, a working group of the WHO, UNICEF, and the World Bank, which has made extensive progress in childhood immunization throughout the world.

I went to Harvard to get a master's degree in tropical public health, then worked in Africa at a medical center. While in Africa, CDC asked me to become involved in the smallpox program in Nigeria. The Nigerian-Biafran civil war broke out in 1967, and I went back to CDC for what I thought would be a few months until the war was over. It stretched on for years. During that time I became involved in smallpox eradication. Once the war was over, I was so obsessed with smallpox eradication that I continued working in that, first in West Africa and then in India.

With smallpox, the real problem was to define where the virus was, so that instead of concentrating wholly on vaccinating people, we were going to get to a point where herd immunity would stop the disease. We found instead that with smallpox you can mark every person who has it because there isn't any real subclinical infection. If a person gets smallpox, they're going to get noticeably sick. We could become much more efficient if we started watching the trail of smallpox, finding the people who were sick, and then trying to vaccinate those exposed to sick people. In a period of weeks, we could stop an outbreak. We tried that in West Africa. It worked so well that even in India, with a high population density, we were able to go from the highest rates that India had had for decades to zero twelve months later. It really was an efficient and fast way to change the whole smallpox battle.

Polio is quite different in that for every clinical case, you may have as many as a thousand subclinical cases, so that virus is going all over. You just see it every once in a while. The principles are still that you try to figure out where is the virus, and you try to put your attention on protecting people in that area. The specifics turn out to be different. With polio, you have to do entire geographic areas over and over, but the principle of tracking still holds up. With polio we can actually fingerprint the virus. I recall so vividly more than twenty-five years ago the first time we could do that. It was with an outbreak in the United States, which happened to be in an Amish community. We were able to fingerprint the virus, track it as it went into different states. We were able to track it back to a religious community in Canada to a religious community in the Netherlands to the Middle East.

One lesson we have learned is that we really do have to think through strategy. A second lesson is the absolute importance of surveillance in disease eradication control. Knowledge is power; we found this out in smallpox. You have to outwit nature by knowing as much as you can know, and surveillance becomes crucial. A third very important lesson is when we do eradication programs, we have to be asking all the time how is this improving the infrastructure that will remain after this disease is gone. We become such zealots, focused on one disease, that we're almost willing to sacrifice other things in order to get that one disease eliminated. With a little more planning and forethought, we could be building the infrastructure for what comes next. We're shortsighted in that regard. Another lesson is that it is possible to get the whole world to agree on things that have to do with health. Health is a universal value that you can use, and we should figure out how to use it as a surrogate for alien invasion; that is, something we all fear and therefore are willing to work together to try to solve.

Bob Keegan has worked at the CDC for more than thirty years. He is a manager who does "double duty" as a technical consultant on some of the polio eradication projects.

I help to coordinate all of CDC's funding, staffing, political issues and partnership issues, so that means managing a staff of about 100 people. We have a budget of about 150 million dollars, and we have relationships with the World Health Organization, UNICEF, Rotary International, and numerous other partners. As part of the polio eradication project, I'm a technical consultant who travels overseas frequently, working with the World Health Organization and Ministries of Health to strengthen their polio eradication efforts.

I'm helping to plan and implement National Immunization Days, to manage surveillance activities in a country, to get additional resources in countries, to manage limited resources most efficiently so we can eradicate polio faster.

I serve as the liaison at CDC with Rotary International, and I'm also a key liaison to UNICEF and to the World Health Organization. That means meeting with their leadership, trying to get joint positions on documents. I am working on an Op Ed piece for the *New York Times* and other newspapers which will be jointly signed by CDC, WHO, UNICEF, and Rotary International. This level of partnership for polio eradication has probably exceeded that for any other public health project both in the scope of activities and its ability to work together effectively.

Early on we had a severe shortage of funding and didn't really think big enough. We didn't really know what it would take to get the job done. The job was presented to us and to the world in 1988. People saw another smallpox eradication program, and it was anything but that. It was much more challenging because we needed more doses of vaccine; the surveillance was more difficult because polio is largely a silent disease; there were far more countries involved; the world is a much more dangerous place in the nineties and 2000s than it was in the 1960s and seventies. It just took so much more money than we'd ever imagined. It's been quite expensive by comparison with previous public health projects, so fundraising became a big part of this.

We've learned the value of political support. I'd place a real value on the partnerships. This partnership has brought together the leadership. We recognize the value, through the partnership, of political support, and the use of partnerships where everybody's approaching the same political leaders to get results.

Previously, you were lucky if you had a political leader involved in something. The Polio Eradication Initiative has the personal engagement of dozens of heads of state, from the President of the United States to the President of France, to the President of Nigeria, the Prime Minister of India, to major states involved personally in the polio program one way or the other. The partnerships help to give us access to political leadership in a way that we've never seen before. Getting people to work together in the different partner organizations has allowed us greater access than if we had just been working by ourselves.

Certainly that partnership helped to raise more funds. This project has raised several billion dollars, and that's unprecedented in the history of public health, certainly at the time that we raised it. The AIDS program may be approaching those kinds of dollars now, but certainly this partnership with polio set the stage for that.

We also learned about the operations of working in difficult countries, everything from ceasefires for children to get them vaccinated, to the very daunting challenges of reaching every child in the most remote locations. It's been a real challenge, but one which we've relished and which we've largely succeeded.

Carol Pandak is the manager of Rotary's PolioPlus Program in Illinois.

I have been involved in polio eradication, first as a supervisor in Rotary International's Polio Plus Program, which is our effort to immunize all the children of the world against polio, and then as the manager of the program. We have Rotary Clubs in over 165 countries, so we have representation on the ground in almost all the countries where polio is a problem, especially West and Central Africa. Almost all the countries that are going to be doing immunization activities over the next two months, twenty-three countries have Rotary Club members. From our headquarters office in Evanston, we work directly with the Rotarians in those particular countries.

Rotary Club members tend to be the business and community leaders; they have access to many of the political leaders, and other influential members of the community who can promote the goal of the Polio Eradication Program. Rotary can very effectively work at the grassroots level, even though we're headquartered here in Evanston.

When I go to Africa, in some countries, on every single corner there are polio victims. In the United States, you never see a polio victim, or very rarely you see an older person. Where polio is still a problem, it's so prevalent that it's almost invisible. They don't even take notice because it's common. Children or teens dragging themselves along the street and begging on the corners—it's a common sight.

I was in India at a polio reconstructive surgery hospital. Some of these kids can't even sit up. They have polio of the spine, and I'd never seen that before. You often see it in the limbs. One of the doctors was talking to the parents who want their children to walk. The guy says, "I'm going to make your child sit up, and by sitting up, your child can sit in school. I will never make your child walk." It's a miracle he can do that.

Anna Rubin is the education and outreach coordinator for the International Reha-
bilitation Center for Polio at Spaulding Rehabilitation Hospital in Massachusetts.

It was my work with polio survivors that inspired me to go to India for a National Immunization Day. I joined a group of Rotarians who were going to northern India. The first day we did sightseeing. In New Delhi, at many of the tourist attractions, just outside the gate or the compound was the first time that I saw what's known as a crawler. A crawler is somebody who can't walk because of polio, and they get around on these flat wooden boards that have wheels on them. At the side of our bus as we were getting out to see a sight, there would be a crawler who would roll over and beg.

My whole reason for going to India and my interest in being there was the notion that I could actually put two drops of polio vaccine onto a child's tongue and thereby insure that that child would never have polio. We were all wearing yellow shirts that said India Polio NID, which means National Immunization Day. The leader of our group said those yellow shirts and your white faces speak volumes. It means a lot to these people that you have come on your own time, on your own means, to be here and that you're committed to eradicating polio. After we went into these little villages to give polio drops, we were supposed to go back again to the same area and do what's called "mop up" work; you go door to door, and ask how many children live there, and ask to see their purple pinkies. Every child who is immunized, their pinky fingernail on their left hand is painted purple, either with a ginshen violet, which is a natural dye, or a purple magic marker. We were supposed to make sure that every child under five had a purple pinky, and if not, we were to give them drops right then and there.

Virginia Swezy is a public health advisor and STOP [Stop Transmission of Polio] team leader at the CDC [Centers for Disease Control and Prevention].

I have been involved with the Polio Eradication Program for nearly seven years, and came on board when the STOP program was just beginning. Since that time I have been working to help support the STOP program and to lead the program. The STOP team program is the initiation of the program at the field level. It's the consultants working in the field for three months at a time. I do two things. I work with colleagues in the field to identify what their gaps are, and I try to identify consultants that can help. I am also traveling to the field and working in surveillance activities as well as supporting Immunization Day activities.

I've learned that a program like this would certainly not be possible without an enormous amount of commitment, dedication, and an incredible partner-ship. It's really been quite remarkable to see this global partnership come together and really achieve this amazing goal.

There are many hurdles that we're confronting daily. Countries have been doing this for quite some time now, so there is some fatigue on the part of the countries to continue to do this. Conducting National Immunization Days is an enormous undertaking. It requires enormous amounts of resources, personnel, funds. If you're doing it over and over again, countries are getting tired.

Some countries haven't seen a case of polio for one or more years, and it's quite difficult to convince them to keep up surveillance. Trying to keep the motivation going can be part of our challenge.

Surveillance is done basically from the grassroots-level up. We depend on the communities as well as the local health facilities to make surveillance systems work. If a child in a community becomes paralyzed, there would be no way at the national level to know about that unless that local grassroots facility is actually reporting it. It requires that local clinic identifying the child and having that local clinic actually report to the central level in the country, and then the central level reporting back to the national level.

Bill Sergeant is a Rotarian who heads the International PolioPlus Committee, a group that was set up by the trustees of the Rotary Foundation of Rotary International to give direction and control and assistance to the PolioPlus Program.

The "Plus" name was applied to it because we envisioned that in addition to immunizing children against polio, we would also be immunizing children against other vaccine-preventable diseases. While the Polio Eradication Initiative did have an important impact on other vaccine-preventable diseases, we did not do what we thought we might be doing when we embarked on the program. We have devoted our primary time, most of our funds and other efforts solely to polio.

Today we have identified other things that perhaps the "Plus" turned out to be. The most important aspect of the "Plus" has been the creation of a laboratory system and a surveillance system, which can be used in the case of other diseases. The laboratories also have the ability to identify and isolate other viruses; therefore, it might turn out to be an important legacy.

We did find that in South America the number of measles cases, while we were immunizing against polio, went down in excess of 90 percent because the populace became sensitive and interested in getting children immunized against other diseases, even though that was not a direct matter to which we applied ourselves.

We were primarily going after polio, but we would probably immunize children against other diseases. It didn't work out that way because use of a needle and the task of keeping clean needles without harming someone. In fact, trying to do that with needles really doesn't work out very well with a vaccine that's being given by mouth and easily applied. There's a certain amount of counter productiveness in trying to combine at an immunization point, particularly in places in Asia and Africa. It did have an indirect and important event, because it alerted the populace. It was part of the education of the people about the importance of immunizing against other diseases. We found it had an impact, although it wasn't as direct as we imagined.

In 1994 the trustees of the foundation decided to set up an International PolioPlus Committee and give it total direction of Rotary's effort; delegated some authority to them; and composed what they felt was a very strong committee. I was selected to chair that committee. I was frankly very reluctant at first, but did agree to do it, and subsequently I've been reappointed every year. I'm now in my eleventh year as chairman, and I'm devoting myself virtually 100 percent to polio.

I work on it every day, and I travel. I've boarded an airplane a hundred times in a year, and I go to various places, various meetings, and other activities of the Polio Eradication Initiative. It's become the biggest part of my life. This is not a paid job; I do this for nothing. Although my expenses are covered, I don't draw any remuneration.

William E. Sprague, M.D., is an obstetrician/gynecologist who has volunteered on international medical missions to more than nineteen countries in thirty-seven years.

I became involved in polio eradication out of my experiences in World War II as a medical corpsman and then combat. I felt that killing people was a bad way to solve problems, so in 1962, after finishing medical school and my residency, I decided every year I would devote three or four weeks to international health.

I was a Rotarian in 1987 when the PolioPlus Project began. I had worked on polio wards and had some of my friends, when I was a youngster, come down with polio. I thought, "This is something I really would want to get involved in." I contacted the PolioPlus manager in Evanston, Illinois, headquarters of Rotary International, and told him that I would like to get involved with this.

A few months later I was on my way to the small countries of the South Pacific to evaluate the presence or absence of polio and the vaccination rates. I went to the Cook Islands, Tonga, Fiji, the Solomon Islands and Guadalcanal. Then I went over to Papua, New Guinea.

When I returned to Grand Rapids, I sent in the report to the PolioPlus manager. He asked me if I would become part of the active polio eradication team for Rotary International. Then I went to China, Vietnam, Cambodia, Thailand. I stayed with the Western Pacific region of polio eradication until we were down to zero cases in that area.

When we went to Afghanistan, at every village, we'd meet with the mullah first. The Taliban was quite active there. He would give us these beads and bless us. I never saw any mistrust when I was in Afghanistan. Our mission there was to eradicate polio.

My most concerning experience was in Somalia, which was 1998. It was all run by warlords. Every area you went to, you had to pay a bribe to go to that particular section. Every place we went, we always had a pickup loaded with soldiers with machine guns behind us to protect us.

One time in southern Somalia, we were going to a small village to immunize their children. We saw a group of soldiers coming up this dirt road. They all had AK-47s. They stopped us; looked in our windows. These soldiers were all thirteen, fourteen, fifteen years of age. The UNICEF person thought, "Well, this is going to be the end of us." Our interpreter, who was the mayor of one of the villages we were going to, talked for about an hour and a half to impress them what our journey was for, but they wouldn't let us proceed. Since we were primarily westerners, they made us turn around and go back, so we never did get down to that area. It's still a very dangerous country to work in.

NOTES

INTRODUCTION

1. John R. Paul, *A History of Poliomyelitis* (New Haven, CT: Yale University Press, 1971), 10–23.

2. Dorothy M. Horstmann, "The Clinical Epidemiology of Poliomyelitis," *Annals of Internal Medicine* 43 (1955), 527–528.

3. Paul, *History of Poliomyelitis*, 79–102, 107–125.

4. Ibid., 107.

5. Naomi Rogers, *Dirt and Disease: Polio before FDR* (New Brunswick, NJ: Rutgers University Press, 1990), 10–11, and passim.

6. Paul, *History of Poliomyelitis*, 159.

7. Rogers, *Dirt and Disease*, 165.

8. The best sources on Roosevelt's polio and its impact on his life and career are Hugh Gregory Gallagher, *FDR's Splendid Deception*, rev. ed. (Arlington, VA: Vandamere Press, 1994); Richard Thayer Goldberg, *The Making of Franklin D. Roosevelt: Triumph over Disability* (Cambridge, MA: Abt Books, 1981); and Geoffrey C. Ward, *A First-Class Temperament: The Emergence of Franklin Roosevelt* (New York: Harper and Row, 1989).

9. Gallagher in *FDR's Splendid Deception* deals extensively with how and why Roosevelt's disability was concealed.

10. Ward, *First-Class Temperament*, 704–754; Gallagher, *FDR's Splendid Deception*, 34–58; and Turnley Walker, *Roosevelt and the Warm Spring Story* (New York: A. A. Wyn, 1953).

11. Daniel J. Wilson, "A Crippling Fear: Experiencing Polio in the Era of FDR," *The Bulletin of the History of Medicine* 72 (1998), 464–495; Amy L. Fairchild, "The Polio Narratives: Dialogues with FDR," *The Bulletin of the History of Medicine* 75 (2001), 488–534.

12. Paul, *History of Poliomyelitis*, 304–323; Richard Carter, *The Gentle Legions* (Garden City, NY: Doubleday, 1961), 91–138; David M. Oshinsky, *Polio: An American Story* (New York: Oxford University Press, 2005), 53–55.

13. Hart E. Van Riper, "Aims, Program, and Achievements of National Foundation for Infantile Paralysis," *JAMA* 157 (January 8, 1955), 141.

14. David J. Rothman, *Beginnings Count: The Technological Imperative in American Health Care*, A Twentieth Century Fund Book (New York: Oxford University Press, 1997), 44–45, 50, 63.

15. Paul, *History of Poliomyelitis*, 339–344.

16. Frederick C. Robbins and Thomas M. Daniel, "A History of Poliomyelitis," in *Polio*, ed. Thomas M. Daniel and Frederick C. Robbins (Rochester, NY: University of Rochester Press, 1997), 15.

17. Paul, *History of Poliomyelitis*, 418.

18. Oshinsky, *Polio*, 188–213.

19. Jane S. Smith, *Patenting the Sun: Polio and the Salk Vaccine* (New York: William Morrow, 1990), 321–322.

20. Paul, *History of Poliomyelitis*, 433–438; Smith, *Patenting the Sun*, 359–367; Oshinsky, *Polio*, 214–236; Paul A. Offitt, *The Cutter Incident: How America's First Polio Vaccine Led to the Growing Vaccine Crisis* (New Haven, CT: Yale University Press, 2005).

21. Paul, *History of Poliomyelitis*, 451.

22. Ibid., 449–456.

23. Bureau of the Census, *Historical Statistics of the United States: Colonial Times to 1970*, 2 vols. (Washington, DC: Government Printing Office, 1975), 1:77; "Incidence Rates of Poliomyelitis in the USA," *Polio Network News* 15 (Fall 1999), 3; Neal Nathanson, "Eradication of Poliomyelitis in the United States," *Reviews of Poliomyelitis in the United States* 4 (1982), 940; "Poliovirus Infections in Four Unvaccinated Children—Minnesota, August–October 2005," *MMWR Dispatch* 54 (October 14, 2005), 1–3.

24. Horstmann, "Clinical Epidemiology of Poliomyelitis," 527–528.

25. In 1940 only 9.3% of the population had hospital insurance and 4.0% had surgical insurance. In 1950 just over half the population (50.7%) had hospital insurance and 35.8% had surgical insurance. Bureau of the Census, *Historical Statistics of the United States*, 1:82.

26. For descriptions of what having polio was like in this period, see Fred Davis, *Passage through Crisis: Polio Victims and Their Families* (1963; reprint, with a new introduction by the author, New Brunswick, NJ: Transaction Publishers, 1991); Kathryn Black, *In the Shadow of Polio: A Personal and Social History* (Reading, MA: Addison-Wesley Publishing Company, 1996); and Daniel J. Wilson, *Living with Polio: The Epidemic and Its Survivors* (Chicago: University of Chicago Press, 2005).

27. Margaret Campbell's survey of 120 polio survivors revealed that only 11% never married, that 49% completed college, and only 3% never worked. Of the 260 polio survivors in the survey by Sandra French and Sam Sloss, 13% never married, 56% had more than a high school education, and 2.7% never worked. Margaret L. Campbell, "'Aging with Polio–101': Risk Factors and Protective Influences?" (paper presented at the Seventh International Post-Polio and Independent Living Conference, St. Louis, MO, May 29, 1997), 3; Sandra S. French and G. Sam Sloss, "Health and Demographic Characteristics of Polio Survivors" (Lincolnshire Post-Polio Library, April 1999, www.ott.zynet.co.uk/polio/lincolnshire/library/usa/kentuckysurvey.htm), 2.

28. David O. Wiechers discovered that the first description of the late effects of poliomyelitis was given by the great French neurologist Jean-Martin Charcot in 1875. He identified twenty-three additional reports from the nineteenth century and ten additional reports and descriptions between 1903 and 1973. David O. Wiechers, "Late Effects of Polio: Historical Perspectives," *Birth Defects Original Article Series* 23 (1987), 1–11.

29. On the role of Gini Laurie and GINI in drawing medical attention to the problems of post-polio syndrome, see Nora Groce, *The U.S. Role in International Disability Activities: A History and a Look Towards the Future* (Oakland: World Institute on Disability, 1992), 150–152; Joan L. Headley, "Independent Living: The Role of Gini Laurie," *Rehabilitation Gazette* 38 (Winter 1998), 1–3.

30. Julie K. Silver, *Post-Polio Syndrome: A Guide for Polio Survivors & Their Families* (New Haven, CT: Yale University Press, 2001); Lauro S. Halstead and Naomi Naierman, eds., *Managing Post-Polio: A Guide to Living Well with Post-Polio Syndrome* (Washington, DC: NRH Press, 1998).

31. Nancy M. Frick, "Post-Polio Sequelae and the Psychology of Second Disability," *Orthopedics* 8 (July 1985), 851–853.

32. Groce, *The U.S. Role in International Disability Activities*, 77–106; Joseph P. Shapiro, *No Pity: People with Disabilities Forging a New Civil Rights Movement* (New York: Times Books/Random House, 1993), 41–73; Doris Zames Fleischer and Frieda Zames, *The Disability Rights Movement: From Charity to Confrontation* (Philadelphia, PA: Temple University Press, 2001), 33–48.

33. Fleischer and Zames, *The Disability Rights Movement*, 149–150.

34. Ibid., 88–109; Shapiro, *No Pity*, 105–141.

35. Oshinsky, *Polio*, 39–50.

36. David L. Sills, *The Volunteers: Means and Ends in a National Organization* (Glencoe, IL: The Free Press, 1957), 25; Carter, *The Gentle Legions*, 110–115; Paul, *History of Poliomyelitis*, 310–311.

37. Paul, *History of Poliomyelitis*, 311; Carter, *The Gentle Legions*, 119–120.

38. Paul, *History of Poliomyelitis*, 318.

39. Van Riper "Aims, Program, and Achievements of National Foundation for Infantile Paralysis," 140.

40. Paul, *History of Poliomyelitis*, 449–450.

41. "Polio Plus: Providing Immunization Worldwide," *AAP [American Academy of Pediatrics] News* (April 1986), 5–6, 10; Chris Anne Raymond, "Worldwide Assault on Poliomyelitis Gathering Support, Garnering Results," *JAMA* 255 (March 28, 1986), 1547.

42. "History of PolioPlus," Rotary International, available at http://www.rotary.org/foundation/polioplus/information/history.htm, accessed July 30, 2003.

43. "Progress Toward Interruption of Wild Poliovirus Transmission—Worldwide, January 2004–March 2005," *MMWR Weekly*, 54 (April 29, 2005), 2 (http://www.cdc.gov/mmwr/preview/mmwrhtml/mm5416a4.htm), accessed December 12, 2005.

44. Rothman, *Beginnings Count*, 42–66.

45. Richard J. McNally, *Remembering Trauma* (Cambridge: Belknap Press of Harvard University Press, 2003), 2, 35, 37, 39, 58, 60.

46. Anne Hunsaker Hawkins, *Reconstructing Illness: Studies in Pathography* (West Lafayette, IN: Purdue University Press, 1993), 14–15.

47. Arthur W. Frank, *The Wounded Storyteller: Body, Illness, and Ethics* (Chicago: University of Chicago Press, 1995), 22, 63.

CHAPTER 1

1. John R. Paul, *A History of Poliomyelitis* (New Haven, CT: Yale University Press, 1971), 79–81, 107.

2. Ibid., 89, 108.

3. Naomi Rogers, *Dirt and Disease: Polio Before FDR* (New Brunswick, NJ: Rutgers University Press, 1990), 10–11, 13–14, 26.

4. Ibid., 14–15.

5. Sheila M. Rothman, *Living in the Shadow of Death: Tuberculosis and the Social Experience of Illness in American History* (New York: Basic Books, 1994), 248; *Historical Statistics of the United States: Colonial Times to 1970*, 2 vols. (Washington, DC: Government Printing Office, 1975), 1:77.

6. *Historical Statistics,* 1:77.

7. Alfred W. Crosby, *America's Forgotten Pandemic: The Influenza of 1918*, 2nd ed. (Cambridge: Cambridge University Press, 2003), 206–207.

8. On Roosevelt, his polio, and its affect on his life and career, see Geoffrey C. Ward, *A First-Class Temperament: The Emergence of Franklin Roosevelt* (New York: Harper and Row, 1989); Hugh Gregory Gallagher, *FDR's Splendid Deception*, rev. ed. (Arlington, VA: Vandamere Press, 1994); and Richard Thayer Goldberg, *The Making of Franklin D. Roosevelt: Triumph over Disability* (Cambridge, MA: Abt Books, 1981).

9. Rogers, *Dirt and Disease,* 166.

10. Paul, *A History of Poliomyelitis,* 212–224.

11. Daniel J. Wilson, "A Crippling Fear: Experiencing Polio in the Era of FDR," *Bulletin of the History of Medicine* 72 (1998), 464–495.

12. Paul, *A History of Poliomyelitis,* 305–306.

13. Ibid., 252–262; quotation on p. 259.

14. David Oshinsky, *Polio: An American Story* (New York: Oxford University Press, 2005), 52–55.

15. Paul, *A History of Poliomyelitis,* 311, 310.

16. Ibid., 311; emphasis in original.

17. David J. Rothman, *Beginnings Count: The Technological Imperative in American Health Care*, A Twentieth Century Fund Book (New York: Oxford University Press, 1997), 42–66; Paul, *A History of Poliomyelitis,* 324–334.

18. Paul, *History of Poliomyelitis,* 344.

19. Dorothy M. Horstmann, "The Clinical Epidemiology of Poliomyelitis," *Annals of Internal Medicine* 43 (1955), 531–532.

20. Neal Nathanson and John R. Martin, "The Epidemiology of Poliomyelitis: Enigmas Surrounding Its Appearance, Epidemicity, and Disappearance," *American Journal of Epidemiology* 110 (1979), 676.

21. Quoted in Fred Davis, *Passage through Crisis: Polio Victims and Their Families* (1963: reprint, with a new introduction by the author, New Brunswick, NJ: Transaction Publishers, 1991), 41.

22. Ibid.

23. "Incidence Rates of Poliomyelitis in the USA," *Polio Network News* 15 (Fall 1999), 3.

CHAPTER 2

1. *Definitive and Differential Diagnosis of Poliomyelitis* (New York: The National Foundation for Infantile Paralysis, 1954); Robert Britt, Amos Christie, and Randolph Batson, "Pitfalls in the Diagnosis of Poliomyelitis," *JAMA* 154 (April 24, 1954), 1401–1403; Irvine McQuarrie, "The Evolution of Signs and Symptoms of Poliomyelitis," in *Poliomyelitis: Papers and Discussions Presented at the First International Poliomyelitis Conference* (Philadelphia: J. B. Lippincott, 1949), 57–61; and John A. Anderson,

"Diagnosis and Treatment of Poliomyelitis in the Early Stage," in *Poliomyelitis: Papers and Discussions Presented at the First International Poliomyelitis Conference*, 109–118.

2. On the segregation of medical treatment and hospitals, see W. Montague Cobb, "Medical Care for Minority Groups," *The Annals of the American Academy of Political and Social Science* 273 (January 1951), 169–175; and Max Seham, "Discrimination against Negroes in Hospitals," *New England Journal of Medicine* 271 (October 29, 1964), 940–943. On the designation of polio hospitals, see "How Hospitals Fought Chicago's Polio Threat," *Hospitals* 30 (1956), 43; and Herbert J. Kaufmann, "The Impact of the 1955 Poliomyelitis Outbreak on the Boston City Hospital," *The Boston Medical Quarterly* 7 (March 1956), 4–5.

3. Thomas M. Daniel, "Polio and the Making of a Doctor," in *Polio*, ed. Thomas M. Daniel and Frederick C. Robbins (Rochester, NY: University of Rochester Press, 1997), 81.

4. For a physician's perspective on the lumbar puncture, see Daniel, "Polio and the Making of a Doctor," 82.

5. Kaufmann, "The Impact of the 1955 Poliomyelitis Outbreak on the Boston City Hospital," 7; Robert S. Marshall, "Polio Epidemic Hits Massachusetts," *Hospitals* 29 (1955), 148, 150.

6. Dorothy M. Horstmann, "The Clinical Epidemiology of Poliomyelitis," *Annals of Internal Medicine* 43 (1955), 532.

7. John Ruhräh and Erwin E. Mayer, *Poliomyelitis in All Its Aspects* (Philadelphia, PA: Lea & Febiger, 1917), 164–166.

8. John R. Paul, *A History of Poliomyelitis* (New Haven, CT: Yale University Press, 1971), 344.

9. Joint Orthopedic Nursing Advisory Service, *Nursing for the Poliomyelitis Patient*, (New York: National Organization for Public Health Nursing and National League of Nursing Education, 1948), 29–37; Elizabeth Kenny, *Treatment of Infantile Paralysis in the Acute Stage* (Minneapolis, MN: Bruce Publishing Company, 1941), 64–79.

10. David J. Rothman, *Beginnings Count: The Technological Imperative in American Health Care,* A Twentieth Century Fund Book (New York: Oxford University Press, 1997), 43–50, quotation on p. 52.

11. Lynne Dunphy, "'Constant and Relentless': The Nursing Care of Patients in Iron Lungs, 1928–1955," in *Nursing Research: A Qualitative Perspective*, 3rd ed., ed. Patricia L. Munhall (Sudbury, MA: Jones and Bartlett Publishers, 2001), 417–438.

12. William T. Green, "The Management of Poliomyelitis: The Convalescent Stage," in *Poliomyelitis: Papers and Discussions Presented at the First International Poliomyelitis Conference*, 165, 169.

13. Ibid., 172.

14. Ibid., 177–181, quotation on p. 181.

15. Rothman, *Beginnings Count*, 63.

16. Joint Orthopedic Nursing Advisory Service, *Nursing for the Poliomyelitis Patient*, 59–61; Kathryn Black, *In the Shadow of Polio: A Personal and Social History* (Reading, MA: Addison-Wesley Publishing Company, 1966), 117–121.

17. Joseph S. Barr, "The Management of Poliomyelitis: The Late Stage," in *Poliomyelitis: Papers and Discussion Presented at the First International Poliomyelitis Conference*, 201–219.

CHAPTER 3

1. David L. Sills, *The Volunteers: Means and Ends in a National Organization* (Glencoe, IL: The Free Press, 1957), 118–124.

2. Fred Davis, *Passage through Crisis: Polio Victims and Their Families* (1963: reprint, with a new introduction by the author, New Brunswick, NJ: Transaction Publishers, 1991), 32, 36–38.

3. See, for example, James Carroll, *An American Requiem: God, My Father, and the War That Came between Us* (Boston, MA: Houghton Mifflin, 1996), 43–48.

4. Davis, *Passage through Crisis*, 40–41.

5. Naomi Rogers, *Dirt and Disease: Polio before FDR* (New Brunswick, NJ: Rutgers University Press, 1990), 33–42.

6. Dorothy M. Horstmann, "The Clinical Epidemiology of Poliomyelitis," *Annals of Internal Medicine* 43 (1955), 528.

7. Davis, *Passage through Crisis*, 38, 42.

8. Herbert J. Kaufmann, "The Impact of the 1955 Poliomyelitis Outbreak on the Boston City Hospital," *Boston Medical Quarterly* 7 (March 1956), 7; Robert S. Marshall, "Polio Epidemic Hits Massachusetts," *Hospitals* 29 (1955), 148; Kathryn Black, *In the Shadow of Polio: A Personal and Social History* (Reading, MA: Addison-Wesley Publishing Company, 1966), 66–70.

9. Davis, *Passage through Crisis*, 58–64, 68.

10. Daniel J. Wilson, "A Crippling Fear: Experiencing Polio in the Era of FDR," *Bulletin of the History of Medicine* 72 (1998), 483–484; Black, *In the Shadow of Polio*, 100–101.

11. U.S. Department of Commerce, Bureau of the Census, *Historical Statistics of the United States: Colonial Times to 1970*, Part 1 (Washington, DC: Government Printing Office, 1975), 82, 164.

12. Sills, *The Volunteers*, 131–132, 135.

13. William T. Green, "The Management of Poliomyelitis: The Convalescent Stage," in *Poliomyelitis: Papers and Discussions Presented at the First International Poliomyelitis Conference* (Philadelphia, PA: J. B. Lippincott Company, 1949), 182.

14. Davis, *Passage through Crisis*, 128–134.

15. Kathryn Black explores the different ways families coped when a parent contracted polio: *In the Shadow of Polio*, see especially 205–206, 251–254.

16. Davis, *Passage through Crisis*, 83–99.

CHAPTER 4

1. For a study of the challenges of living with polio, see Daniel J. Wilson, *Living with Polio: The Epidemic and Its Survivors* (Chicago: University of Chicago Press, 2005).

2. Margaret L. Campbell, "Aging with Polio—101: Risk Factors and Protective Influences," paper presented at the *Seventh International Post-Polio and Independent Living Conference*, St. Louis, May 29, 1997, 3; Sandra S. French and G. Sam Sloss, "Health and Demographic Characteristics of Polio Survivors" (A Lincolnshire Post-Polio Library Publication, April 1999), available at http://www.ott.zynet.co.uk/polio/lincolnshire/library/usa/kentuckysurvey.htm, p. 2.

3. On domestic life and the baby boom in the postwar years, see Elaine Tyler May, *Homeward Bound: American Families in the Cold War Era* (New York: Basic Books,

1988), 3–9, 159–161; Steven Mintz and Susan Kellogg, *Domestic Revolution: A Social History of American Family Life* (New York: The Free Press, 1988), 177–201.

4. Recent surveys of polio survivors suggest that between 10 and 15% of them never married. Campbell, "Aging with Polio–101," 3; French and Sloss, "Health and Demographic Characteristics of Polio Survivors," 2; Richard L. Bruno and Nancy M. Frick, "The Psychology of Polio as Prelude to Post-Polio Sequelae: Behavior Modification and Psychotherapy," *Orthopedics* 14 (November 1991), 1188.

5. May, *Homeward Bound*, 5–8.

CHAPTER 5

1. David L. Sills, *The Volunteers: Means and Ends in a National Organization* (Glencoe, IL: The Free Press, 1957), 8.

2. Geoffrey C. Ward, *A First-Class Temperament: The Emergence of Franklin Roosevelt* (New York: Harper & Row, 1989), 770; Turnley Walker, *Roosevelt and the Warm Springs Story* (New York: A. A. Wyn, 1953), 143.

3. Tony Gould, *A Summer Plague: Polio and Its Survivors* (New Haven, CT: Yale University Press, 1995), 45, 54–57, 60–63; David M. Oshinsky, *Polio: An American Story* (New York: Oxford University Press, 2005), 47–53.

4. Gould, *A Summer Plague*, 73–74; Oshinsky, *Polio*, 53–55.

5. Sills, *The Volunteers*, 21, 25, 28, 70.

6. John R. Paul, *A History of Poliomyelitis* (New Haven, CT: Yale University Press, 1971), 312.

7. Sills, *The Volunteers*, 85–86.

8. Ibid., 95–96.

9. Ibid., 99–100.

10. Ibid., 30–31.

11. Ibid., 149, 154–162.

12. Doris Zames Fleischer and Frieda Zames, *The Disability Rights Movement: From Charity to Confrontation* (Philadelphia, PA: Temple University Press, 2001), 71–76, 82–86.

13. Nora Groce, *The U.S. Role in International Disability Activities: A History and a Look Towards the Future* (New York and Oakland, CA: World Institute on Disability, World Rehabilitation Fund, and Rehabilitation International, 1992), 150–152; Gazette International Networking Institute, "History of Organization," http://www.post-polio.org/hist.html (accessed July 28, 2003); Joan L. Headley, "Independent Living: The Role of Gini Laurie," *Rehabilitation Gazette* 38 (Winter 1998), 1–3.

14. Jonathan Majiyagbe, "The Volunteers' Contribution to Polio Eradication," *Bulletin of the World Health Organization* 82 (January 2004), 2; Daniel Tarantola, "PAHO at the Forefront of Immunization and Disease Elimination," *American Journal of Public Health* 92 (December 2002), 1886.

15. Gustav J. V. Nossal, "Gates, GAVI, the Glorious Global Funds and More: All You Ever Wanted to Know," *Immunology and Cell Biology* 81 (2003), 21.

CHAPTER 6

1. Daniel J. Wilson, "A Crippling Fear: Experiencing Polio in the Era of FDR," *Bulletin of the History of Medicine* 72 (1998), 464–495.

2. John Duffy, "Franklin Roosevelt Ambiguous Symbol for Disabled Americans," *Midwest Quarterly* 29 (1987), 113.

3. Amy Fairchild, "The Polio Narratives: Dialogues with FDR," *Bulletin of the History of Medicine* 75 (2001), 500, 515.

4. Irving Kenneth Zola, *Missing Pieces: A Chronicle of Living with a Disability* (Philadelphia, PA: Temple University Press, 1982), 203–205.

5. Paul K. Longmore and David Goldberger, "The League of the Physically Handicapped and the Great Depression: A Case Study in the New Disability History," in Paul K. Longmore, *Why I Burned My Book and Other Essays on Disability* (Philadelphia, PA: Temple University Press, 2003), 63.

6. Ibid., 65–70

7. Ibid., 84.

8. Ibid., 57. There is also an account of the League of the Physically Handicapped in Doris Zames Fleischer and Frieda Zames, *The Disability Rights Movement: From Charity to Confrontation* (Philadelphia, PA: Temple University Press, 2001), 5–7.

9. Joseph P. Shapiro, *No Pity: People with Disabilities Forging a New Civil Rights Movement* (New York: Times Books, 1993), 41–45.

10. Ibid., 50–51.

11. Ibid., 53–55.

12. Ibid., 55–58.

13. Interview with Kathryn Vastyshak by Daniel J. Wilson, Allentown, PA, June 25, 2002.

14. Fleischer and Zames, *The Disability Rights Movement*, 149; Shapiro, *No Pity*, 71; "Ronald L. Mace, 1941–1998," Biographical Note, Ronald Mace Collection, Special Collections, North Carolina State University Libraries, Raleigh, NC, accessed at www.lib.ncsu.edu/archives/collections/html/mace_mc260.html (July 28, 2003).

15. Hugh Gregory Gallagher, *Black Bird Fly Away: Disabled in an Able-Bodied World* (Arlington, VA: Vandamere Press, 1998), 107–109.

16. Fred Fay and Fred Pelka, "Justin Dart, an Obituary," accessed at www.aapd-dc.org/docs/jdanobituary.html (July 28, 2003); Fleischer and Zames, *The Disability Rights Movement*, 88–93.

CHAPTER 7

1. David O. Wiechers, "Late Effects of Polio: Historical Perspectives," *Birth Defects Original Articles Series* 23 (1987), 1, 3, 5–7. Wiechers found ten case reports between 1903 and 1973 and nine from 1962 to 1986.

2. Lori J. Klein, *Post-Polio Syndrome: January 1967 through September 1989*, Current Bibliographies in Medicine (Bethesda, MD: National Library of Medicine, 1989) and search of the National Library of Medicine's online bibliography, *PubMed*, August 2004.

3. Gertrud Weiss, "Gini and G.I.N.I. Conferences: Pioneering Independent Living," *Polio Network News* 9 (Fall 1993), 1–2; Joan Headley, "Independent Living: The Role of Gini Laurie," *Rehabilitation Gazette* 38 (Winter 1998), 1–3; Nora Groce, *The U.S. Role in International Disability Activities: A History and a Look Towards the Future* (Oakland, CA: The World Institute on Disability, The World Rehabilitation Fund, and Rehabilitation International, 1992), 150–152.

4. Frederick M. Maynard and Joan L. Headley, ed., *Handbook on the Late Effects of Poliomyelitis for Physicians and Survivors*, rev. ed. (Saint Louis, MO: Gazette International

Networking Institute, 1999); Lauro Halstead and Naomi Naierman, eds., *Managing Post-Polio: A Guide to Living Well with Post-Polio Syndrome* (Washington, DC: NRH Press, 1998); Julie K. Silver, *Post-Polio: A Guide for Polio Survivors & Their Families* (New Haven, CT: Yale University Press, 2001); *March of Dimes International Conference on Post-Polio Syndrome: Identifying Best Practices in Diagnosis and Care* (White Plains, NY: The March of Dimes Birth Defects Foundation, 2001).

5. Silver, *Post-Polio*, 17.

6. Ibid., 18.

7. Ibid., 21–26. In any epidemic, over 90% of those infected showed no symptoms or paralysis. Dorothy M. Horstmann, "The Clinical Epidemiology of Poliomyelitis," *Annals of Internal Medicine* 43 (1955), 528.

8. See note 4.

9. Carol J. Gill, "Overcoming Overcoming," in Halstead and Naierman, *Managing Post-Polio*, 208–209; Silver, *Post-Polio*, 249–254.

CHAPTER 8

1. See, for example, Daniel J. Wilson, *Living with Polio: The Epidemic and Its Survivors* (Chicago: University of Chicago Press, 2005); David M. Oshinsky, *Polio: An American Story* (New York: Oxford University Press, 2005); Marc Shell, *Polio and Its Aftermath: The Paralysis of Culture* (Cambridge: Harvard University Press, 2005); Jeffrey Kluger, *Splendid Solution: Jonas Salk and the Conquest of Polio* (New York: G. P. Putnam's Sons, 2004); *A Paralyzing Fear: The Story of Polio in America*, VHS, directed by Nina Gilden Seavey (Washington, DC: PBS Video, 1998); and *A Fight to the Finish: Stories of Polio*, VHS, directed by Ken Mandel (Dallas, TX: Texas Scottish Rite Hospital for Children/Ken Mandel Productions, 1999).

2. John R. Paul, *A History of Poliomyelitis* (New Haven, CT: Yale University Press, 1971), 374–376.

3. "Infantile Paralysis: Pioneers in Treatment," *Physical Therapy*, 56 (January 1976), 42–43; see also Jay Schleichkorn, "Physical Therapist, 98, Recalls Rehabilitating Franklin Roosevelt," *P. T. Bulletin* (March 16, 1988), 24–27.

4. "The Beginning of 'Modern Physiotherapy,'" *Physical Therapy* 56 (January 1976), 15–18.

5. Donald A. Neumann, "Polio: Its Impact on the People of the United States and the Emerging Profession of Physical Therapy," *Journal of Orthopedic & Sports Physical Therapy* 34 (August 2004), 479.

6. Hugh Gregory Gallagher, *FDR's Splendid Deception*, rev. ed. (Arlington, VA: Vandamere Press, 1994), 53–56; Paul, *A History of Poliomyelitis*, 302; Schleichkorn, "Physical Therapist, 98," 24–27.

7. David J. Rothman, *Beginnings Count: The Technological Imperative in American Health Care*, A Twentieth Century Fund Book (New York: Oxford, 1997), 42–48.

8. Ibid., 51, 58.

9. Ibid., 63–64; Robert M. Eiben, "The Polio Experience and the Twilight of the Contagious Disease Hospital," in *Polio*, ed. Thomas M. Daniel and Frederick C. Robbins (Rochester, NY: University of Rochester Press, 1997), 108–110; and Kathryn Black, *In the Shadow of Polio: A Personal and Social History* (Reading, MA: Addison-Wesley Publishing Company, 1996).

10. Roxanne Nelson, "On Borrowed Time," *AARP Bulletin* (September 2004), 20.

11. Jessie Wright, "Factors Related to Prescription in Poliomyelitis, " *The Physiotherapy Review* 27 (July/August 1947), 229.

12. Chris Anne Raymond, "Polio Survivors Spurred Rehabilitation Advances," *JAMA* 255 (March 21, 1986), 1403; Nina Gilden Seavey, Jane S. Smith, and Paul Wagner, *A Paralyzing Fear: The Triumph over Polio* (New York: TV Books, 1998), 141–142.

13. Raymond, "Polio Survivors," 1403; Rothman, *Beginnings Count*, 113–114.

14. Raymond, "Polio Survivors," 1403–1404.

15. Hart E. Van Riper, "Aims, Program, and Achievements of National Foundation for Infantile Paralysis," *JAMA* 157 (January 8, 1955), 142; Kimberly Ferren Carter, "Trumpets of Attack: Collaborative Efforts between Nursing and Philanthropies to Care for the Child Cripples with Polio 1930 to 1959," *Public Health Nursing* 18 (July/August 2001), 253, 256–257, 259.

16. Donald S. Burke, "Lessons Learned from the 1954 Field Trial of Poliomyelitis Vaccine," *Clinical Trials* 1 (2004), 3–5.

17. Lawrence K. Altman, "Health Officials Say They'll End Polio in Africa, Despite Its Spread," *New York Times*, January 16, 2005, 9.

18. Technical Consultative Group to the World Health Organization on the Global Eradication of Poliomyelitis, "'Endgame' Issues for the Global Polio Eradication Initiative," *Clinical Infectious Disease* 34 (2002), 72–75.

19. D. A. Henderson, "Countering the Posteradication Threat of Smallpox and Polio," *Clinical Infectious Diseases* 34 (2002), 80, 82–83.

20. Technical Consultative Group, "Endgame," 74.

INDEX

Acute and convalescent polio
  early years, 42–43
  1930s, 43
  1940s, 43–47
  1950s, 47–56
  1960s and after, 57
Acute paralytic poliomyelitis, 6, 37
ADAPT (American Disabled for
  Accessible Public Transit), 98
African Americans and civil rights, 111
Americans, contracted with paralytic
  polio, 1
Americans with Disabilities Act (ADA)
  (1990), 10, 98, 114–15
Attenuated live polio vaccine, 5

Bill and Melinda Gates Foundation, 99
Brodie, Maurice, 16
Burke, Donald, 143
Bush, George H.W., 115

Camp Greentop, 23
Cantor, Eddie, 17
Carnevale, Peter, 148
Caverly, Charles S., 15
Center for Independent Living (CIL), 113
Coping behavior, post-polio syndrome,
  126–27
  Abbot, Noreen, 137
  Arnold, Dorothy, 136
  Esau, Ruth, 136
  Givant, Kathleen, 137

Lappin, Judy, 136
O'Connor, Edward, 135–36
Schweid, Bill, 135
Vickery, Margo, 135
Zanke, William, 134–35
Cutter incident, 32

Daniel, Thomas, 35
Dart, Justin, Jr., 10, 115
Davis, Fred, 59
Disability Awareness Day, 117
Disability Movement, 86, 117–18
Disabled in Action (DIA), 98, 114
Disabled Students Program, 117–18
Drinker, Philip, 3, 37, 141
"Drinker" respirator, 30
Duffy, John, 111

Enders, John, 4
Epidemic years, of polio, 140
  beginning of mass vaccination, 19
  care and therapeutic methods, 17–18
  cases of unsuccessful human trials, 16
  characteristics in the forties and fifties,
    18–19
  early years (1916–1929), 19
  establishment of NFIP, 17, 141
  hospital admissions, 35–39
  Kenny's methods of treatment, 18
  in Los Angeles (1934), 16
  in New York (1907 and 1916),
    15–16

Epidemic Years(*cont.*)
   1930s, 20
   1940s, 21–24
   1950s, 24–32
   1960s and after, 32–33
   summer of 1894, 15

Fairchild, Amy, 111
Family responses, to polio, 7
   Durr, George, 131
   early years, 63
   financial strain, 61
   hospital discharge, 62
   hospitalization impacts, 60–61
   Kellogg, Ted, 133
   1930s, 63–65
   1940s, 65–68
   1950s, 68–73
   1960s, 73–74
   parental guilt feelings, 59
   Pierce, Mike, 131–32
   public health quarantines, 59–60
   Rosenwald, Richard, 130–31
   Zanke, William, 131
Federal Architectural Barriers Act
   (1968), 115
Flexner, Simon, 2
Foege, William, 149–50
Francis, Thomas, Jr., 4
Frank, Arthur, 12

Gallagher, Hugh, 115
Gazette International Networking
   Institute (GINI), 9, 99
Georgia Warm Springs Foundation, 3,
   10, 40, 95–96, 140
Green, William, 39

Hawkins, Anne Hunsaker, 12
Henderson, Donald, 143
Heumann, Judy, 98, 114–15
Horstmann, Dorothy, 18

Independent Living Movement, 119
Influenza epidemic of 1918–1919, 16
Iron lungs, 3, 17–18, 20, 37–38, 141

Jack Martin Polio Respirator Center,
   29

Keegan, Bob, 150–51
Kenny, Sister Elizabeth, 4, 17, 37
Kenny hot packs, 6–7
Killed-virus vaccine, 4–5
Kolmer, John A., 16

Landsteiner, Karl, 2, 15
Laurie, Gini, 9
The League of the Physically
   Handicapped, 112
Lehigh Valley Center for Independent
   Living, 114
Life experiences after polio, early years
   DiBona, Anthony, 19
   Esau, Ruth, 42–43, 63
   Piageri, Pearl, 19
   Taylor, Ray, 147–48
Life experiences after polio, 1930s
   Cote, Alice, 43, 63–64, 81
   Drinker, Philip, 20
   Durr, George, 65, 81–82
   Emerson, John Haven, 20
   Huse, Robert, 79–81
   Lang, Bernice, 20
   Lonardo, Robert, 78
   Rubin, David, 79
   Rugh, Joan, 63
Life experiences after polio, 1940s
   Balber, Ellen, 66–67
   Barrett, Diana, 24
   Brewer, Everlene, 84–85
   Cox, Carol, 84
   Hall, Lucille, 24
   Heumann, Judith Ellen, 85–86
   Hindson, Edna, 47
   Hoffshire, Irja, 23–24
   Jordan, Arlene, 68
   Kellogg, Ted, 22–23, 46, 65–66, 84,
   146
   Kistler, J. Phillip, 43–44
   McKnight, Samuel, 68
   McNally, Frank, 21
   Nau, Beatrice Yvonne, 46–47,
   67
   Norkunas, Bill, 82–83
   Pappas, Katherine, 22, 45–46
   Pierce, Mike, 22, 45
   Schweid, Bill, 44–45
   Spalsbury, Rick, 67–68

Vickery, Margo, 43–44
Yamazaki, James, 21
Zanke, William, 21–22, 83
Life experiences after polio, 1950s
   Alford, Margaret, 51–52
   Alford, Peggy, 90
   Barker, Sylvia M., 29–31
   Berenberg, William, 31
   Bloom, Fred, 70
   Blute, Robert D., 53–54
   Brown, Regina, 55
   Burwick, Stephen, 51
   Charlton, Earl P. "Chuck," 28
   Diamond, Steven, 25–26, 69
   Donahue, Emily, 69, 88–90
   Graceffa, Steffano, 86–87
   Greenberg, Ernest, 56
   Griffin, Jody Leigh, 25, 50–51
   Handal, Ken, 47–48
   Houghton, Priscilla Dewey, 68–69
   Huegel, Vince, 91–92
   Hussey, Ann Lee, 27, 91
   Jackson, Edwina, 55–56
   Liew, Thelma Van, 28–29
   Lubin, Lawrence "Larry," 54–55
   Marshall, Margaret, 52–53
   Masters, Michael, 71–72
   Meehan, Norma, 52, 73, 90–91
   O'Connor, Edward, 25, 49–50,
      72–73, 87
   Rosenwald, Richard, 48–49
   Salk, Jonathan, 31–32
   Smothers, Gloria, 54
   Sternburg, Dottie, 87–88
   Stevens, Margaret Barry, 88
   Thorpe, Philip, 28
   Vance, Mary Lee, 92
   Wells, Neil, 72
   Werner, Ruthanne, 70–71
   Willemy, Judith, 26
   Wills-Foster, Siddequeh, 48
Life experiences after polio, 1960s and
   after
   Alexander, Margaret, 74
   Donohue, Aimee, 92–93
   Donohue, Jean, 93
   Erilus, Ewald, 93
   Guckin, Justine, 32–33, 57, 73–74,
      92, 146

Longmore, Paul, 112
Lovett, Robert, 140

Mace, Ron, 10, 114–15
"March of Dimes and Americans," 10,
   17–18, 95
   Hindson, Edna, 100
   Kennedy, Chester "Chet," 100–101
   management, 97
   volunteer membership, 97–98
Massage and Therapeutic Exercise, 140
McMillan, Mary, 140
McNally, Richard J., 12

National Foundation for Infantile
   Paralysis (NFIP), 1, 3–4, 9–11, 17,
      38, 95, 139, 141
   fundings, 142
   management, 97
   volunteer membership, 97–98
National Immunization Day, 104, 106

O'Connor, Basil, 10, 17, 95, 143
Odhner, Carl, 114–15
Operation Overcome, 114

Pan American Health Organization,
   99
Pandak, Carol, 152
Paralysis, treatment of, 4
Parental guilt feelings and polio, 59
People of Color Movement, 118
Physically Disabled Students Program
   (PDSP), 113
Plastridge, Alice Lou, 140
Polio
   in ancient world, 1–2
   case of Roosevelt, F. D., 3
   client experiences, 6
   convalescence from, 39
   development of other devices, 142
   development of respirators, 142
   diagnostic procedures, 35–36
   discovery of virus, 2
   distinction between spinal and bulbar
      polio, 38
   epidemic statistics, 2, 5
   etiology, 2
   families of adult polio patients, 7

Polio(*cont.*)
   locations of therapy, 40
   post-polio syndrome, 9
   rehabilitation methods, 40–42
   rehabilitation and protestant work
      ethic, 8
   survivors, 3–4, 8–10
   and treatment of paralysis, 4
   and use of iron lungs, 141
   vaccine development, 4–5, 143
   as a weapon of bioterrorism, 143
Poliomyelitis, 1, 6, 23
Polio Oral History Project, 6, 11
Polio Pioneer Extraordinary, 100
PolioPlus program, 11
Polio Voices, 11–12
Popper, Erwin, 2, 15
Post-Polio Health International, 95
Post-polio syndrome, 9
   and advocacy efforts of polio
      survivors, 124–25
   coping, 126–27
   criteria for diagnosis, 126
   etiology, 125
   Guckin, Justine, 129–30
   impact on families, 125–27
   Kellogg, Ted, 129
   O'Connor, Edward, 128–29
   problems of polio survivors,
      125
   Schweid, Bill, 129
   symptoms, 123–24
   treatment planning, 126
   Vickery, Margo, 127–28
Protestant work ethic and polio
   rehabilitation, 8

Quality of life, after polio
   Burwick, Stephen, 134
   Griffin, Jody Leigh, 133
   Guckin, Justine, 133–34

Reagan, Ronald, 115
Rehabilitation Gazette, 98–99
Remembering Trauma, 12
Respiratory assistive devices, 30,
   142
Robbins, Frederick, 4
Roberts, Ed, 98, 113, 115

Rocking bed, 17, 87
Rogers, Naomi, 15–16
Roosevelt, Franklin D., 3, 9, 16, 95–96,
   111, 140
Rotary International, 11, 99
   Groner, David, 101–4
   Hussey, Ann Lee, 106–7
   Sergeant, Bill, 153–54
   Serra, Joseph, 107–8
   Youlton, Terry, 104–6
Rothman, David, 38, 142
Rubin, Anna, 152–53

Sabin, Albert, 5, 21, 32
Sabin vaccine, 1, 11, 19, 95, 100,
   118
Salk, Jonas, 4
Salk vaccine, 1, 4–5, 11, 19, 30, 95,
   100, 143
Silver, Julie, 126, 128
Sprague, William E., 154–55
Summer flu, 25
Survivors, of polio
   disability rights movement, 111–15
   Faye, Fred, 120–21
   Headley, Joan, 119–20
   Heumann, Judith Ellen, 116–18
   Hindson, Edna, 116
   job openings, 77–78
   The League of the Physically
      Handicapped, 112
   Lonardo, Robert, 120
   mainstreaming of, 112
   1930s, 78–82
   1940s, 82–86
   1950s, 86–92
   1960s and after, 92–93
   resilience, 75
   Roberts, Ed, 113–14
   as students, 76–77
Swezy, Virginia, 153

Universal design, for disabled people,
   114

Volunteerism, 9, 11
   contributions, 99
   efforts of Laurie, Virginia (Gini),
      98–99

establishment of NFIP, 95–96
President's Birthday Ball Commission, 95–96
support groups, 99

Weller, Thomas, 4
Whelan, John Patrick, 143–46

Works Progress Administration (WPA) program, 112
World Health Organization (WHO), 1, 99
  Aylward, Bruce, 108–9, 148–49

Zola, Irving Kenneth, 111

About the Authors

JULIE SILVER, M.D., is Assistant Professor at Harvard Medical School and the Medical Director of the International Rehabilitation Center for Polio (IRCP) at Spaulding Rehabilitation Hospital. A world-renowned expert on post-polio syndrome, she has published widely with seven authored books and eight edited collections to her credit, as well as dozens of articles in peer-reviewed journals, magazines, and newspapers. She is the author of *Post-Polio Syndrome: A Guide for Polio Survivors and Their Families*, which received the Will Solimene Award of Excellence from the American Medical Writers Association. Silver is also Series Editor for two Praeger series, Contemporary Health and Wellness, and Rehabilitation and Recovery after Injury or Disease. For more information regarding polio, her polio books, or the IRCP, visit www.polioclinic.org.

DANIEL WILSON, Ph.D., has been teaching history of medicine for more than a decade and is Professor of History at Muhlenberg College. He was a Fellow with the Agency of Healthcare Research and Quality National Endowment for the Humanities. He has given presentations on the polio epidemics at meetings of the American Association for the History of Medicine, The American Historical Association, and the International Post-Polio and Independent Living Conference, as well as at Harvard University and Columbia University. Wilson is, himself, a polio survivor.